INSPIRATIONAL STORIES OF RESILIENCE AND FIGHT

LIGHT IN SHADOWS

BY

VISHNU S KUMAR

INTRODUCTION

THE COVID-19 PANDEMIC SWEPT ACROSS THE GLOBE, LEAVING IN ITS WAKE A TRAIL OF HEARTBREAK, FEAR, AND UNCERTAINTY. IT DESCENDED UPON US SWIFTLY, DISRUPTING LIVES AND SHATTERING OUR SENSE OF NORMALCY. AS THE VIRUS SPREAD RELENTLESSLY, IT UNLEASHED AN UNPRECEDENTED EMOTIONAL STORM THAT ENGULFED INDIVIDUALS AND COMMUNITIES, LEAVING NO ONE UNTOUCHED.

IN THE EARLY DAYS, ANXIETY PERMEATED THE AIR LIKE A HEAVY FOG. FEARFUL WHISPERS

ECHOED THROUGH NEIGHBORHOODS, AS PEOPLE GRAPPLED WITH THE UNKNOWN. THE INVISIBLE THREAT SEEMED TO LURK AROUND EVERY CORNER, TURNING EVEN THE SIMPLEST OF TASKS INTO DAUNTING CHALLENGES. AS THE NUMBER OF INFECTIONS SOARED AND LOVED ONES FELL ILL, THE EMOTIONAL TOLL BECAME UNBEARABLE.

LONELINESS SETTLED LIKE AN UNWELCOME GUEST, AS ISOLATION MEASURES SEVERED THE THREADS THAT BOUND US TOGETHER. FAMILIES WERE TORN APART, UNABLE TO EMBRACE OR SEEK SOLACE IN EACH OTHER'S PRESENCE. THE ELDERLY, ONCE PILLARS OF WISDOM AND STRENGTH, BECAME THE MOST VULNERABLE, CONFINED TO THE ISOLATION OF THEIR HOMES, THEIR EYES LONGING FOR THE WARMTH OF HUMAN CONNECTION.

STUDENTS, USUALLY VIBRANT AND FILLED WITH YOUTHFUL ENTHUSIASM, FOUND THEMSELVES ADRIFT IN A SEA OF UNCERTAINTY. CLASSROOM LAUGHTER WAS REPLACED BY THE FLICKERING GLOW OF COMPUTER SCREENS, AS VIRTUAL

EDUCATION BECAME THE NORM. THE ABSENCE OF CLASSMATES, TEACHERS, AND THE REASSURING STRUCTURE OF SCHOOL LEFT A VOID IN THEIR HEARTS, AND THEIR DREAMS OF GRADUATION AND CELEBRATION TURNED INTO DISTANT MIRAGES.

THE HALLS OF COMMERCE ECHOED WITH THE CRIES OF STRUGGLING BUSINESS. ENTREPRENEURS, FUELED BY THEIR DREAMS, WERE SUDDENLY FACED WITH THE HARSH REALITY OF CLOSURES AND BANKRUPTCY. EMPLOYEES, ONCE THE BACKBONE OF THRIVING ESTABLISHMENTS, FACED JOB LOSSES AND FINANCIAL DESPAIR. THE WEIGHT OF RESPONSIBILITY PRESSED UPON THEIR HEARTS, AS THEY WONDERED HOW THEY WOULD PROVIDE FOR THEIR FAMILIES AND MAKE ENDS MEET.

IN THE REALM OF ART AND ENTERTAINMENT, A DEAFENING SILENCE FELL UPON STAGES, THEATERS, AND MOVIE SETS. THE VIBRANT TAPESTRY OF CULTURE, ONCE ALIVE WITH THE MAGIC OF PERFORMANCES, NOW STOOD EMPTY

AND ABANDONED. MUSICIANS, ACTORS, AND ARTISTS, WHOSE TALENT BROUGHT JOY AND MEANING TO OUR LIVES, FOUND THEMSELVES WITHOUT A PLATFORM TO EXPRESS THEIR CREATIVITY, LEAVING THEIR SOULS YEARNING FOR THE APPLAUSE OF A LIVE AUDIENCE.

AMIDST THESE CHALLENGES, WOMEN AND MEN FACED A DIFFERENT SET OF BURDENS. THE INVISIBLE CHAINS OF GENDER INEQUALITY TIGHTENED AS THE PANDEMIC RAGED ON. WOMEN, OFTEN AT THE FOREFRONT OF CAREGIVING, FOUND THEMSELVES SHOULDERING EVEN HEAVIER LOADS, JUGGLING WORK, HOMESCHOOLING, AND THE EMOTIONAL WELL-BEING OF THEIR FAMILIES. MEN, TOO, GRAPPLED WITH THEIR OWN STRUGGLES, NAVIGATING THE PRESSURES OF PROVIDING AND PROTECTING IN A WORLD TURNED UPSIDE DOWN.

THE STRAIN ON OUR COLLECTIVE PSYCHE REVERBERATED BEYOND THE REALMS OF FINANCE AND HEALTH. THE EMOTIONAL IMPACT SEEPED INTO THE VERY FABRIC OF OUR BEINGS,

LEAVING SCARS THAT MAY TAKE YEARS TO HEAL. YET, AMIDST THE DARKNESS, GLIMMERS OF RESILIENCE AND HOPE EMERGED. COMMUNITIES RALLIED TOGETHER, EXTENDING HELPING HANDS TO THOSE IN NEED. STRANGERS BECAME FRIENDS, CONNECTING THROUGH SHARED EXPERIENCES AND ACTS OF COMPASSION. THE HUMAN SPIRIT, TESTED AND STRAINED, SHOWED ITS INDOMITABLE STRENGTH, REFUSING TO BE DEFEATED.

AS WE EMBARK ON THIS JOURNEY THROUGH THE STRUGGLES, SURVIVAL, AND TRIUMPHS OF THE COMMON MAN DURING THE COVID-19 PANDEMIC, LET US BEAR WITNESS TO THE RAW EMOTIONS THAT HAVE COURSED THROUGH OUR VEINS. TOGETHER, WE SHALL NAVIGATE THE DEPTHS OF DESPAIR AND RISE WITH UNWAVERING DETERMINATION. THIS IS A STORY OF THE TRIUMPH OF THE HUMAN SPIRIT, WHERE LOVE, RESILIENCE, AND THE WILL TO SURVIVE HAVE PERSEVERED AGAINST ALL ODDS.

THE COVID-19 PANDEMIC HAS UNLEASHED A WAVE OF HARDSHIP AND SUFFERING THAT

KNOWS NO BORDERS. IT HAS REMINDED US, IN THE STARKEST OF TERMS, THAT OUR SHARED HUMANITY CONNECTS US ALL. IN EVERY CORNER OF THE WORLD, INDIVIDUALS AND COMMUNITIES HAVE GRAPPLED WITH UNIMAGINABLE CHALLENGES, ENDURING PAIN, LOSS, AND PROFOUND UNCERTAINTY. AS WE EMBARK ON THIS JOURNEY THROUGH THEIR STORIES, LET US EXTEND OUR EMPATHY AND UNDERSTANDING, ACKNOWLEDGING THE IMMENSE BURDEN THEY HAVE CARRIED.

TO THOSE WHO HAVE LOST LOVED ONES, WE STAND WITH YOU IN YOUR GRIEF. THE VOID LEFT BY THEIR ABSENCE IS AN ACHE THAT RESONATES IN THE DEEPEST RECESSES OF THE SOUL. WE UNDERSTAND THE PROFOUND SORROW OF NOT BEING ABLE TO BID FAREWELL, TO HOLD A HAND, OR TO SHARE A FINAL EMBRACE. THE PAIN YOU CARRY IS A TESTAMENT TO THE LOVE AND BONDS THAT WERE WOVEN INTO THE TAPESTRY OF YOUR LIVES.

TO THE BRAVE HEALTHCARE WORKERS, WE OFFER OUR DEEPEST GRATITUDE AND ADMIRATION. YOU HAVE FACED THE RELENTLESS ONSLAUGHT OF THIS VIRUS, STANDING AT THE FRONTLINES, RISKING YOUR OWN WELL-BEING TO CARE FOR OTHERS. YOUR TIRELESS EFFORTS, COUNTLESS SLEEPLESS NIGHTS, AND UNWAVERING DEDICATION HAVE NOT GONE UNNOTICED. WE SEE YOUR SACRIFICES, BOTH VISIBLE AND HIDDEN, AND WE HONOR THE STRENGTH AND COMPASSION THAT CONTINUE TO GUIDE YOUR EVERY ACTION.

TO THE STUDENTS, WHOSE WORLDS HAVE BEEN UPENDED, WE UNDERSTAND YOUR FRUSTRATION AND YEARNING FOR NORMALCY. THE ABSENCE OF SCHOOLMATES, THE LAUGHTER OF THE PLAYGROUND, AND THE JOY OF SHARED LEARNING HAVE LEFT AN EMPTINESS WITHIN YOU. WE ACKNOWLEDGE THE CHALLENGES OF REMOTE EDUCATION, THE LOSS OF MILESTONES, AND THE UNCERTAINTY THAT LOOMS OVER YOUR FUTURE. YOU ARE NOT ALONE IN YOUR

HOPES AND DREAMS; TOGETHER, WE WILL FIND A WAY FORWARD.

TO THE BUSINESS OWNERS AND EMPLOYEES WHO HAVE STRUGGLED TO KEEP LIVELIHOODS INTACT, WE ACKNOWLEDGE THE WEIGHT OF YOUR WORRIES AND THE UNCERTAINTY THAT SHADOWS EACH DAY. THE PRESSURES OF FINANCIAL SURVIVAL, THE SLEEPLESS NIGHTS, AND THE AGONIZING DECISIONS YOU HAVE HAD TO MAKE HAVE TESTED YOUR RESILIENCE. WE RECOGNIZE YOUR TENACITY, YOUR RESOURCEFULNESS, AND YOUR UNWAVERING SPIRIT IN THE FACE OF ADVERSITY.

TO THE ARTISTS AND ENTERTAINERS, WHOSE PASSION IS THE LIFEBLOOD OF OUR CULTURAL LANDSCAPE, WE FEEL YOUR PAIN AND MOURN THE LOSS OF STAGES THAT ONCE BURST WITH ENERGY AND CREATIVITY. THE SILENCE THAT HAS SETTLED UPON THEATERS, GALLERIES, AND CONCERT HALLS IS A PROFOUND LOSS FOR US ALL. WE UNDERSTAND THE YEARNING TO SHARE YOUR ART WITH THE WORLD, AND WE

EAGERLY AWAIT THE DAY WHEN YOUR TALENTS WILL ONCE AGAIN GRACE OUR LIVES.

TO EVERYONE WHOSE LIVES HAVE BEEN UPENDED, WHOSE DREAMS HAVE BEEN DEFERRED, AND WHOSE FUTURES HANG IN THE BALANCE, WE HOLD YOUR STRUGGLES CLOSE TO OUR HEARTS. WE ACKNOWLEDGE THE EMOTIONAL TOLL, THE SLEEPLESS NIGHTS, AND THE MOMENTS OF DESPAIR THAT HAVE PUNCTUATED THIS ARDUOUS JOURNEY. YOUR STORIES RESONATE WITH US, REMINDING US THAT BEHIND EVERY STATISTIC LIES A HUMAN FACE, A BEATING HEART, AND A SPIRIT THAT REFUSES TO BE BROKEN.

AS WE DELVE INTO THE NARRATIVES OF THE COMMON MAN'S FIGHT AGAINST COVID-19, LET US CARRY THIS EMPATHY AND UNDERSTANDING AS A GUIDING LIGHT. TOGETHER, MAY WE HONOR THEIR EXPERIENCES, AMPLIFY THEIR VOICES, AND WORK TOWARDS A FUTURE WHERE NO ONE IS LEFT BEHIND.

STRUGGLE AND SURVIVAL OF FAMILIES

JOB LOSS AND FINANCIAL STRUGGLES:

THE PANDEMIC UNLEASHED AN UNPRECEDENTED WAVE OF JOB LOSSES, LEAVING MANY FAMILIES GRAPPLING WITH FINANCIAL HARDSHIPS. BREADWINNERS SUDDENLY FOUND THEMSELVES UNEMPLOYED AS BUSINESSES SHUTTERED, LEADING TO A LOSS OF INCOME AND A SENSE OF UNCERTAINTY ABOUT THE FUTURE. FAMILIES STRUGGLED TO MEET THEIR BASIC NEEDS, SUCH AS PAYING RENT, UTILITIES, AND PUTTING

FOOD ON THE TABLE. THE WEIGHT OF FINANCIAL STRESS WEIGHED HEAVILY ON THEIR SHOULDERS, OFTEN RESULTING IN DIFFICULT DECISIONS AND SACRIFICES.

REMOTE LEARNING CHALLENGES:

THE TRANSITION TO REMOTE LEARNING PRESENTED SIGNIFICANT CHALLENGES FOR FAMILIES. PARENTS HAD TO ADAPT TO NEW ROLES AS EDUCATORS, TRYING TO SUPPORT THEIR CHILDREN'S EDUCATION WHILE MANAGING THEIR OWN WORK RESPONSIBILITIES. LIMITED ACCESS TO TECHNOLOGY AND INTERNET CONNECTIVITY POSED ADDITIONAL BARRIERS, PARTICULARLY FOR FAMILIES FROM DISADVANTAGED BACKGROUNDS. STUDENTS FACED DIFFICULTIES IN STAYING ENGAGED, COPING WITH THE ABSENCE OF FACE-TO-FACE INTERACTION, AND GRAPPLING WITH THE DIGITAL DIVIDE.

HEALTH CONCERNS AND FEAR OF INFECTION:

FAMILIES EXPERIENCED HEIGHTENED HEALTH CONCERNS AND FEARS OF CONTRACTING THE VIRUS. THE CONSTANT WORRY FOR THE WELL-BEING OF FAMILY MEMBERS, ESPECIALLY THOSE WHO WERE MORE VULNERABLE, SUCH AS THE ELDERLY OR THOSE WITH UNDERLYING HEALTH CONDITIONS, CREATED A PERVASIVE SENSE OF ANXIETY. FAMILIES HAD TO NAVIGATE SAFETY PROTOCOLS, SOCIAL DISTANCING MEASURES, AND THE EMOTIONAL TOLL OF BEING SEPARATED FROM LOVED ONES TO MITIGATE THE RISK OF INFECTION.

MENTAL HEALTH STRUGGLES:

THE PANDEMIC TOOK A TOLL ON THE MENTAL HEALTH OF INDIVIDUALS AND FAMILIES. THE STRESSORS OF JOB LOSS, FINANCIAL STRAIN, SOCIAL ISOLATION, AND HEALTH CONCERNS LED TO INCREASED LEVELS OF ANXIETY, DEPRESSION, AND FEELINGS OF HELPLESSNESS. FAMILIES HAD TO GRAPPLE WITH THE EMOTIONAL IMPACT OF THE PANDEMIC, BALANCING THEIR OWN WELL-BEING WHILE PROVIDING SUPPORT TO THEIR LOVED ONES. ACCESS TO MENTAL HEALTH RESOURCES AND SERVICES BECAME CRUCIAL BUT OFTEN LIMITED.

STRAINS ON RELATIONSHIPS:

THE PROLONGED CONFINEMENT AND HEIGHTENED STRESS PUT STRAINS ON FAMILY RELATIONSHIPS. SPENDING EXTENSIVE TIME TOGETHER UNDER ONE ROOF, WITH LIMITED SOCIAL

INTERACTIONS OUTSIDE THE HOUSEHOLD, TESTED PATIENCE AND COMMUNICATION SKILLS. COUPLES FACED CHALLENGES IN BALANCING WORK, HOUSEHOLD RESPONSIBILITIES, AND CHILD-REARING. SIBLINGS EXPERIENCED CONFLICTS ARISING FROM SHARED SPACES AND DISRUPTED ROUTINES. THE INABILITY TO CONNECT WITH EXTENDED FAMILY AND FRIENDS ADDED TO A SENSE OF ISOLATION AND LONELINESS.

THESE DIFFICULTIES ILLUMINATE THE MULTIFACETED STRUGGLES FAMILIES FACED DURING THE PANDEMIC. THE COMPOUNDING EFFECTS OF JOB LOSS, REMOTE LEARNING CHALLENGES, HEALTH CONCERNS, MENTAL HEALTH STRAINS, AND RELATIONSHIP PRESSURES MADE NAVIGATING DAILY LIFE EXCEPTIONALLY CHALLENGING. HOWEVER, FAMILIES DEMONSTRATED RESILIENCE, ADAPTABILITY, AND THE POWER OF COMING TOGETHER TO SUPPORT ONE ANOTHER THROUGH THESE UNPRECEDENTED TIMES.

THE RODRIGUEZ FAMILY:

THE RODRIGUEZ FAMILY CONSISTED OF THREE GENERATIONS LIVING UNDER ONE ROOF. THEY WERE A CLOSE-KNIT FAMILY THAT RELIED ON EACH OTHER FOR SUPPORT AND STRENGTH. WHEN THE PANDEMIC STRUCK, THEY WERE DEVASTATED BY THE LOSS OF THEIR BELOVED GRANDMOTHER, A PILLAR OF THEIR FAMILY. THE LOSS WAS NOT ONLY EMOTIONALLY CHALLENGING BUT ALSO HIGHLIGHTED THE FRAGILITY OF LIFE AND THE IMPORTANCE OF CHERISHING THEIR BOND.

AMID THE GRIEF, THE FAMILY ALSO FACED FINANCIAL HARDSHIPS. BOTH PARENTS LOST THEIR JOBS AS THE ECONOMY TOOK A HIT. THEY STRUGGLED TO MAKE ENDS MEET AND WORRIED ABOUT HOW THEY WOULD PROVIDE FOR THEIR CHILDREN AND MAINTAIN STABILITY IN THEIR LIVES. THE WEIGHT OF THEIR FINANCIAL BURDENS THREATENED TO TEAR THEM APART.

HOWEVER, THE RODRIGUEZ FAMILY REFUSED TO LET ADVERSITY DEFINE THEM. INSTEAD, THEY DREW ON THEIR DEEP LOVE AND DETERMINATION TO KEEP THEIR FAMILY TOGETHER. THEY RECOGNIZED THAT IN TIMES OF CRISIS, THEIR UNITY AND SUPPORT FOR ONE ANOTHER WOULD BE THEIR GREATEST STRENGTH.

THEY RALLIED AROUND EACH OTHER, OFFERING EMOTIONAL SUPPORT AND ENCOURAGEMENT. THEY SHARED THE BURDEN OF FINANCIAL RESPONSIBILITIES, WORKING TOGETHER TO FIND ALTERNATIVE SOURCES OF INCOME AND EXPLORE NEW OPPORTUNITIES.

THEY REMAINED RESILIENT, REMINDING THEMSELVES OF THE STRENGTH THEY DERIVED FROM THEIR SHARED LOVE AND MEMORIES.

THE RODRIGUEZ FAMILY HONORED THEIR GRANDMOTHER'S MEMORY BY PRESERVING THE VALUES SHE HAD INSTILLED IN THEM. THEY EMBRACED HER WISDOM AND RESILIENCE, USING IT AS A GUIDING FORCE TO NAVIGATE THROUGH THE CHALLENGES THEY FACED. THEY FOUND SOLACE IN THEIR SHARED MEMORIES, HOLDING ONTO THE LOVE AND LESSONS SHE HAD IMPARTED.

THROUGH THEIR DETERMINATION, THE RODRIGUEZ FAMILY BEGAN TO REBUILD THEIR LIVES. THEY TAPPED INTO THEIR RESOURCEFULNESS, SEEKING OUT NEW EMPLOYMENT OPPORTUNITIES, ACQUIRING NEW SKILLS, AND LEVERAGING THEIR NETWORKS. THEY WERE UNWAVERING IN THEIR PURSUIT OF STABILITY AND SECURITY FOR THEIR FAMILY.

THE LOVE AND DETERMINATION WITHIN THE RODRIGUEZ FAMILY NOT ONLY HELPED THEM OVERCOME THEIR FINANCIAL STRUGGLES BUT ALSO BROUGHT THEM CLOSER TOGETHER. THEY STRENGTHENED THEIR BOND, FOSTERING AN ENVIRONMENT OF OPEN COMMUNICATION AND SUPPORT. THEY FOUND COMFORT IN KNOWING THAT THEY COULD RELY ON ONE ANOTHER, EVEN IN THE FACE OF ADVERSITY.

THE STORY OF THE RODRIGUEZ FAMILY EXEMPLIFIES THE POWER OF LOVE, DETERMINATION, AND RESILIENCE IN THE FACE OF CHALLENGES. THROUGH THEIR UNITY AND SHARED COMMITMENT, THEY NOT ONLY SURVIVED THE HARDSHIPS OF THE PANDEMIC BUT ALSO EMERGED STRONGER. THEIR STORY SERVES AS AN INSPIRATION, REMINDING US OF THE IMPORTANCE OF FAMILY, LOVE, AND UNWAVERING DETERMINATION IN NAVIGATING DIFFICULT TIMES.

THE CHEN FAMILY :

THE CHEN FAMILY CONSISTED OF PARENTS AND THEIR TWO CHILDREN. THEY WERE A TIGHT-KNIT FAMILY WHO ALWAYS SUPPORTED AND UPLIFTED EACH OTHER. HOWEVER, WHEN THE PANDEMIC HIT, THEY WERE MET WITH UNEXPECTED HARDSHIPS. THE FAMILY'S FINANCIAL SITUATION TOOK A DOWNTURN, FORCING THEIR ELDEST SON TO PUT HIS EDUCATION ON HOLD DUE TO FINANCIAL CONSTRAINTS. THIS SETBACK BROUGHT A WAVE OF DISAPPOINTMENT AND WORRY TO THE FAMILY.

DESPITE THE DIFFICULTIES, THE CHEN FAMILY REFUSED TO LET THESE CHALLENGES DEFINE THEM. THEIR LOVE FOR ONE ANOTHER AND THEIR UNWAVERING DETERMINATION BECAME

THE DRIVING FORCE THAT KEPT THEM UNITED AND MOTIVATED TO FIND SOLUTIONS.

THEY RECOGNIZED THE IMPORTANCE OF EDUCATION FOR THEIR CHILDREN'S FUTURE AND WERE DETERMINED TO PROVIDE THEM WITH THE BEST OPPORTUNITIES. THE PARENTS IMMEDIATELY SPRANG INTO ACTION, SEARCHING FOR ALTERNATIVE WAYS TO SUPPORT THEIR SON'S EDUCATION WHILE MANAGING THEIR FINANCIAL CONSTRAINTS. THEY EXPLORED SCHOLARSHIPS, GRANTS, AND OTHER FORMS OF FINANCIAL AID TO HELP ALLEVIATE THE BURDEN.

SIMULTANEOUSLY, THE CHEN FAMILY EMBRACED A POSITIVE ATTITUDE AND CREATED A

STRUCTURED ROUTINE AT HOME. THEY ESTABLISHED A DEDICATED SPACE FOR STUDYING, ENSURING THAT THEIR CHILDREN HAD AN ENVIRONMENT CONDUCIVE TO LEARNING. THEY TOOK TURNS PROVIDING GUIDANCE AND SUPPORT, MAKING SURE THEIR ELDEST SON HAD THE NECESSARY RESOURCES AND ENCOURAGEMENT TO CONTINUE HIS EDUCATION OUTSIDE OF THE TRADITIONAL CLASSROOM SETTING.

FURTHERMORE, THE CHEN FAMILY LEVERAGED THE POWER OF THEIR LOVE AND DETERMINATION TO OVERCOME FINANCIAL OBSTACLES. THEY CUT BACK ON UNNECESSARY EXPENSES, MADE SACRIFICES, AND TAPPED INTO THEIR RESOURCEFULNESS TO FIND CREATIVE

WAYS TO GENERATE INCOME. THEY EXPLORED NEW SKILLS AND PURSUED SIDE JOBS TO SUPPLEMENT THEIR FINANCES. THE ENTIRE FAMILY CONTRIBUTED, WORKING TOGETHER AS A TEAM, AND CELEBRATING EVEN THE SMALLEST VICTORIES ALONG THE WAY.

THROUGH THEIR UNWAVERING LOVE AND DETERMINATION, THE CHEN FAMILY INSPIRED AND UPLIFTED ONE ANOTHER. THEY MOTIVATED EACH OTHER TO STAY FOCUSED AND PERSEVERE, REMINDING THEMSELVES THAT THEIR UNITY WAS THE KEY TO OVERCOMING OBSTACLES. THEIR LOVE ACTED AS A CONSTANT SOURCE OF ENCOURAGEMENT, REMINDING THEM OF THEIR COLLECTIVE GOAL TO PROVIDE A BETTER FUTURE FOR THEIR CHILDREN.

THE CHEN FAMILY'S STORY IS A TESTAMENT TO THE POWER OF LOVE, DETERMINATION, AND RESILIENCE IN THE FACE OF ADVERSITY. THEIR UNWAVERING COMMITMENT TO SUPPORTING EACH OTHER AND THEIR CHILDREN'S EDUCATION SHOWCASES THE STRENGTH THAT CAN BE FOUND WITHIN A CLOSE-KNIT FAMILY. BY HARNESSING THEIR LOVE AND DETERMINATION, THEY WERE ABLE TO NAVIGATE THE CHALLENGES OF THE PANDEMIC AND CREATE A PATH FORWARD, DEMONSTRATING THAT WITH A STRONG FAMILY BOND, ANYTHING IS POSSIBLE.

THE JOHNSON FAMILY:

THE JOHNSON FAMILY CONSISTED OF PARENTS AND THEIR TWO CHILDREN. THEY WERE A LOVING AND CLOSE-KNIT FAMILY WHO VALUED TOGETHERNESS AND SUPPORT. WHEN THE PANDEMIC STRUCK, THEY FACED MULTIPLE CHALLENGES THAT TESTED THEIR STRENGTH AND RESILIENCE. HOWEVER, THEIR LOVE AND DETERMINATION TO OVERCOME THESE OBSTACLES KEPT THEM UNITED.

ONE OF THE MAJOR CHALLENGES THE JOHNSON FAMILY FACED WAS THE LOSS OF THEIR JOBS AND FINANCIAL INSTABILITY. THE SUDDEN JOB LOSS PUT A SIGNIFICANT STRAIN ON THEIR FINANCES, LEAVING THEM UNCERTAIN ABOUT HOW THEY WOULD PROVIDE FOR THEIR FAMILY'S NEEDS. DESPITE THIS SETBACK, THEY REFUSED TO LET DESPAIR TAKE HOLD.

INSTEAD, THE JOHNSON FAMILY TURNED TO THEIR UNWAVERING LOVE FOR EACH OTHER AS A SOURCE OF MOTIVATION AND SUPPORT. THEY HELD FAMILY MEETINGS TO DISCUSS THEIR SITUATION OPENLY AND TRANSPARENTLY, FOSTERING AN ENVIRONMENT OF TRUST AND OPEN COMMUNICATION. THEY REASSURED ONE

ANOTHER THAT THEY WERE IN THIS TOGETHER AND WOULD FIND A WAY FORWARD.

WITH DETERMINATION, THE JOHNSON FAMILY EMBARKED ON A JOURNEY OF RESILIENCE AND ADAPTATION. THEY EXPLORED NEW AVENUES FOR EMPLOYMENT, INCLUDING REMOTE WORK OPPORTUNITIES AND ONLINE BUSINESSES. THEY HONED THEIR SKILLS, EMBRACED ENTREPRENEURSHIP, AND SUPPORTED EACH OTHER'S ENDEAVORS. THEY BECAME A SOURCE OF INSPIRATION FOR ONE ANOTHER, REMINDING THEMSELVES OF THEIR COLLECTIVE STRENGTH AND THE POWER OF THEIR UNITY.

ADDITIONALLY, THE JOHNSON FAMILY SOUGHT SUPPORT FROM THEIR EXTENDED NETWORK

AND COMMUNITY. THEY CONNECTED WITH OTHER FAMILIES FACING SIMILAR CHALLENGES, SHARING RESOURCES, JOB OPPORTUNITIES, AND EMOTIONAL SUPPORT. THEY REALIZED THAT BY COMING TOGETHER AND SUPPORTING ONE ANOTHER, THEY COULD NAVIGATE THROUGH THE DIFFICULTIES MORE EFFECTIVELY.

MOREOVER, THE JOHNSON FAMILY FACED THE CHALLENGE OF BEING PHYSICALLY SEPARATED FROM THEIR EXTENDED FAMILY AND FRIENDS. THE INABILITY TO GATHER AND SEEK COMFORT IN THE PRESENCE OF LOVED ONES ADDED TO THEIR EMOTIONAL STRAIN. HOWEVER, THEY FOUND INNOVATIVE WAYS TO STAY CONNECTED VIRTUALLY, ORGANIZING REGULAR VIDEO CALLS, VIRTUAL GAME NIGHTS, AND SHARING

STORIES OF HOPE AND RESILIENCE. THEIR DETERMINATION TO STAY EMOTIONALLY CONNECTED DEMONSTRATED THE DEPTH OF THEIR LOVE AND THE LENGTHS THEY WOULD GO TO SUPPORT ONE ANOTHER.

THROUGHOUT THEIR JOURNEY, THE JOHNSON FAMILY'S LOVE AND DETERMINATION REMAINED UNWAVERING. THEY KNEW THAT THEIR UNITY AND SUPPORT WERE PARAMOUNT IN OVERCOMING THE CHALLENGES THEY FACED. THEIR DETERMINATION TO PROVIDE STABILITY AND A NURTURING ENVIRONMENT FOR THEIR CHILDREN FUELED THEIR RESILIENCE. THROUGH THEIR COLLECTIVE EFFORTS AND UNWAVERING LOVE, THEY EMERGED STRONGER, DEMONSTRATING THAT EVEN IN THE FACE OF

ADVERSITY, A UNITED FAMILY CAN FIND THE STRENGTH TO OVERCOME OBSTACLES AND CREATE A SENSE OF HOPE.

THE JOHNSON FAMILY'S STORY SERVES AS A POWERFUL REMINDER OF THE RESILIENCE AND POWER OF LOVE WITHIN A FAMILY. BY STAYING UNITED, SUPPORTING ONE ANOTHER, AND REMAINING DETERMINED, THEY NOT ONLY SURVIVED THE HARDSHIPS OF THE PANDEMIC BUT ALSO FOUND NEW OPPORTUNITIES FOR GROWTH AND STRENGTH.

THE KUMAR FAMILY:

THE KUMAR FAMILY RESIDED IN A RURAL AREA, WHERE THEY OWNED A SMALL FARM. THEY LIVED A SIMPLE LIFE AND HAD A DEEP CONNECTION WITH THEIR LAND, THEIR HERITAGE, AND THEIR COMMUNITY. WHEN THE PANDEMIC STRUCK, THE KUMAR FAMILY FACED A UNIQUE SET OF CHALLENGES THAT THREATENED THEIR WAY OF LIFE.

ONE OF THEIR PRIMARY CONCERNS WAS THE HEALTH AND SAFETY OF THEIR ELDERLY FAMILY MEMBER WHO HAD PRE-EXISTING HEALTH CONDITIONS, MAKING THEM PARTICULARLY VULNERABLE TO COVID-19. THE FAMILY KNEW THAT PROTECTING THEIR LOVED ONE WAS OF UTMOST IMPORTANCE, BUT IT MEANT MAKING

SIGNIFICANT ADJUSTMENTS TO THEIR DAILY LIVES.

TO ENSURE THE SAFETY OF THEIR VULNERABLE FAMILY MEMBER, THE KUMAR FAMILY MADE COLLECTIVE SACRIFICES. THEY STRICTLY ADHERED TO SAFETY PROTOCOLS, INCLUDING LIMITING THEIR INTERACTIONS OUTSIDE THE HOME AND PRACTICING RIGOROUS HYGIENE MEASURES. THEY MAINTAINED A VIGILANT APPROACH, RECOGNIZING THAT THEIR LOVED ONE'S WELL-BEING DEPENDED ON THEIR UNWAVERING COMMITMENT TO SAFETY.

SIMULTANEOUSLY, THE KUMAR FAMILY FACED THE CHALLENGE OF KEEPING THEIR FARM RUNNING WHILE ALSO TAKING CARE OF THEIR

FAMILY'S NEEDS. THEY HAD TO FIND A DELICATE BALANCE BETWEEN MAINTAINING THEIR LIVELIHOOD AND MINIMIZING RISKS. THEY TAPPED INTO THEIR RESOURCEFULNESS AND ADAPTED THEIR FARMING PRACTICES TO ADDRESS THE NEW REALITIES BROUGHT ABOUT BY THE PANDEMIC. THEY EXPLORED ALTERNATIVE METHODS, SUCH AS ONLINE MARKETPLACES AND HOME DELIVERIES, TO ENSURE THEIR PRODUCE REACHED THE COMMUNITY WHILE ADHERING TO SAFETY GUIDELINES.

THROUGHOUT THEIR JOURNEY, THE KUMAR FAMILY'S LOVE AND DETERMINATION WERE PALPABLE. THEY WORKED TOGETHER AS A UNIT, SHARING THE RESPONSIBILITIES AND

SUPPORTING ONE ANOTHER EMOTIONALLY. THEIR DEEP LOVE AND RESPECT FOR THEIR ELDERLY FAMILY MEMBER GAVE THEM THE STRENGTH TO ENDURE THE HARDSHIPS AND MAKE THE NECESSARY SACRIFICES.

DESPITE THE CHALLENGES THEY FACED, THE KUMAR FAMILY FOUND SOLACE IN THEIR SHARED LOVE FOR EACH OTHER AND THEIR COMMUNITY. THEY ACTIVELY SOUGHT SUPPORT FROM THEIR NEIGHBORS AND CONNECTED WITH LOCAL ORGANIZATIONS TO ACCESS ESSENTIAL SUPPLIES AND RESOURCES. THEY REALIZED THAT BY BANDING TOGETHER WITH THEIR COMMUNITY, THEY COULD OVERCOME THE DIFFICULTIES MORE EFFECTIVELY.

THE KUMAR FAMILY'S STORY IS A TESTAMENT TO THE POWER OF LOVE, DETERMINATION, AND COMMUNITY SUPPORT. THEIR UNWAVERING COMMITMENT TO PROTECTING THEIR VULNERABLE FAMILY MEMBER SHOWCASED THE STRENGTH THAT CAN BE FOUND WITHIN A FAMILY BOND. THROUGH THEIR RESILIENCE, ADAPTABILITY, AND DEEP-ROOTED LOVE, THEY DEMONSTRATED THAT EVEN IN THE FACE OF ADVERSITY, A UNITED FAMILY CAN FIND THE STRENGTH TO OVERCOME CHALLENGES AND PRESERVE THEIR WAY OF LIFE.

THE KUMAR FAMILY'S JOURNEY SERVES AS AN INSPIRATION, HIGHLIGHTING THE IMPORTANCE OF FAMILY, LOVE, AND UNWAVERING DETERMINATION IN NAVIGATING DIFFICULT

TIMES. THEIR STORY REMINDS US OF THE POWER OF UNITY AND RESILIENCE, SHOWING THAT THROUGH LOVE AND DETERMINATION, FAMILIES CAN CONFRONT AND TRIUMPH OVER THE CHALLENGES THAT COME THEIR WAY.

THE MARTINEZ FAMILY:

THE MARTINEZ FAMILY WAS A CLOSE-KNIT FAMILY CONSISTING OF PARENTS AND THEIR THREE CHILDREN. THEY LIVED IN A BUSTLING CITY AND ENJOYED A VIBRANT AND ACTIVE LIFESTYLE. HOWEVER, WHEN THE PANDEMIC STRUCK, THEIR LIVES TOOK AN UNEXPECTED

TURN, PRESENTING THEM WITH NUMEROUS CHALLENGES.

ONE OF THE MAJOR CHALLENGES THE MARTINEZ FAMILY FACED WAS THE SUDDEN LOSS OF INCOME. BOTH PARENTS LOST THEIR JOBS DUE TO THE ECONOMIC DOWNTURN CAUSED BY THE PANDEMIC. THE SUDDEN FINANCIAL STRAIN THREATENED THEIR ABILITY TO PROVIDE FOR THEIR CHILDREN AND MAINTAIN THEIR PREVIOUS LIFESTYLE. HOWEVER, THEY REFUSED TO LET DESPAIR OVERWHELM THEM.

INSTEAD, THE MARTINEZ FAMILY DREW STRENGTH FROM THEIR UNWAVERING LOVE AND DETERMINATION TO OVERCOME THESE OBSTACLES. THEY RECOGNIZED THE

IMPORTANCE OF SUPPORTING ONE ANOTHER DURING THESE CHALLENGING TIMES AND FOSTERING A POSITIVE AND RESILIENT MINDSET.

THE PARENTS IMMEDIATELY TOOK ACTION, EXPLORING ALTERNATIVE EMPLOYMENT OPPORTUNITIES AND REEVALUATING THEIR BUDGET TO MAKE ENDS MEET. THEY SOUGHT SUPPORT FROM GOVERNMENT PROGRAMS, COMMUNITY ORGANIZATIONS, AND LOCAL JOB PLACEMENT SERVICES. THEIR DETERMINATION TO PROVIDE FOR THEIR CHILDREN FUELED THEIR RESILIENCE, PUSHING THEM TO EXPLORE NEW CAREER PATHS AND ACQUIRE NEW SKILLS.

THE MARTINEZ FAMILY ALSO FACED THE CHALLENGE OF ADJUSTING TO REMOTE LEARNING FOR THEIR CHILDREN. WITH SCHOOLS TRANSITIONING TO ONLINE PLATFORMS, THEY HAD TO CREATE A CONDUCIVE LEARNING ENVIRONMENT AT HOME WHILE JUGGLING THEIR OWN WORK RESPONSIBILITIES. THEY TRANSFORMED THEIR LIVING SPACE INTO A DESIGNATED STUDY AREA, ENSURING THEIR CHILDREN HAD THE NECESSARY RESOURCES AND SUPPORT TO CONTINUE THEIR EDUCATION.

FURTHERMORE, THE MARTINEZ FAMILY LEANED ON THEIR LOVE FOR ONE ANOTHER TO NAVIGATE THE EMOTIONAL CHALLENGES BROUGHT BY THE PANDEMIC. THEY FOSTERED

OPEN COMMUNICATION, ENCOURAGING EACH FAMILY MEMBER TO EXPRESS THEIR FEELINGS AND CONCERNS. THEY OFFERED SUPPORT AND COMFORT, REMINDING EACH OTHER THAT THEY WERE IN THIS TOGETHER.

DESPITE THE DIFFICULTIES THEY FACED, THE MARTINEZ FAMILY DISCOVERED NEW STRENGTHS AND OPPORTUNITIES ALONG THE WAY. THEY FOUND SOLACE IN THEIR SHARED ACTIVITIES, SUCH AS COOKING TOGETHER, ENGAGING IN INDOOR EXERCISES, AND PURSUING HOBBIES AS A FAMILY. THEY EMBRACED THE OPPORTUNITY TO SPEND QUALITY TIME TOGETHER, STRENGTHENING THEIR BOND AND CREATING LASTING MEMORIES.

THROUGH THEIR LOVE AND DETERMINATION, THE MARTINEZ FAMILY DEMONSTRATED RESILIENCE AND ADAPTABILITY. THEY TRANSFORMED SETBACKS INTO OPPORTUNITIES FOR GROWTH AND REMAINED UNITED IN THE FACE OF ADVERSITY. THEIR UNWAVERING COMMITMENT TO SUPPORTING ONE ANOTHER AND THEIR BELIEF IN A BRIGHTER FUTURE ALLOWED THEM TO PERSEVERE.

THE MARTINEZ FAMILY'S STORY IS A TESTAMENT TO THE POWER OF LOVE, DETERMINATION, AND RESILIENCE IN THE FACE OF CHALLENGES. DESPITE THE FINANCIAL STRAIN, EDUCATIONAL ADJUSTMENTS, AND EMOTIONAL TOLL, THEY FOUND STRENGTH WITHIN THEIR FAMILY BOND. THEIR STORY SERVES AS AN INSPIRATION,

REMINDING US THAT THROUGH LOVE AND DETERMINATION, FAMILIES CAN NAVIGATE DIFFICULT TIMES, ADAPT TO NEW CIRCUMSTANCES, AND EMERGE STRONGER TOGETHER.

THE LEE FAMILY:

THE LEE FAMILY CONSISTED OF PARENTS AND THEIR TWO CHILDREN. THEY WERE A TIGHT-KNIT FAMILY WITH A DEEP BOND AND A SHARED COMMITMENT TO SUPPORTING ONE ANOTHER. WHEN THE PANDEMIC STRUCK, THEY

FACED A MYRIAD OF CHALLENGES THAT TESTED THEIR RESILIENCE AND STRENGTH.

ONE OF THE MAJOR CHALLENGES THE LEE FAMILY ENCOUNTERED WAS THE SUDDEN LOSS OF EMPLOYMENT FOR BOTH PARENTS. THE ABRUPT HALT IN THEIR INCOME CREATED FINANCIAL UNCERTAINTIES, THREATENING THEIR ABILITY TO PROVIDE FOR THEIR CHILDREN AND MAINTAIN STABILITY IN THEIR LIVES. HOWEVER, THEY REFUSED TO LET DESPAIR CONSUME THEM.

DRIVEN BY THEIR UNWAVERING LOVE AND DETERMINATION, THE LEE FAMILY EMBARKED ON A JOURNEY OF ADAPTATION AND RESOURCEFULNESS. THEY RECOGNIZED THE

IMPORTANCE OF SUPPORTING ONE ANOTHER DURING THIS TRYING TIME AND EXPLORED NEW AVENUES FOR EMPLOYMENT AND FINANCIAL STABILITY. THEY SOUGHT OUT JOB OPPORTUNITIES IN DIFFERENT SECTORS AND ACQUIRED NEW SKILLS TO INCREASE THEIR MARKETABILITY.

THE LEE FAMILY'S RESILIENCE EXTENDED BEYOND FINANCIAL CONCERNS. THEY ALSO FACED THE CHALLENGE OF ADJUSTING TO REMOTE LEARNING FOR THEIR CHILDREN. WITH SCHOOLS TRANSITIONING TO ONLINE PLATFORMS, THEY HAD TO CREATE A CONDUCIVE LEARNING ENVIRONMENT AT HOME WHILE BALANCING THEIR OWN WORK RESPONSIBILITIES. THEY EMBRACED THE ROLE

OF FACILITATORS, PROVIDING GUIDANCE AND SUPPORT TO THEIR CHILDREN'S EDUCATIONAL PURSUITS.

FURTHERMORE, THE LEE FAMILY PRIORITIZED THEIR MENTAL AND EMOTIONAL WELL-BEING. THEY ACKNOWLEDGED THE STRESS AND ANXIETY THAT THE PANDEMIC BROUGHT AND ACTIVELY ENGAGED IN ACTIVITIES TO NURTURE THEIR MENTAL HEALTH. THEY PRACTICED OPEN COMMUNICATION, CREATING A SAFE SPACE FOR EACH FAMILY MEMBER TO EXPRESS THEIR FEELINGS AND CONCERNS. THEY SOUGHT SOLACE IN SHARED ACTIVITIES, SUCH AS OUTDOOR WALKS, FAMILY GAME NIGHTS, AND CREATIVE PROJECTS.

THROUGH THEIR UNWAVERING LOVE AND DETERMINATION, THE LEE FAMILY FOUND STRENGTH AND RESILIENCE. THEY INSPIRED AND SUPPORTED ONE ANOTHER, REMINDING THEMSELVES THAT THEY WERE IN THIS TOGETHER. THEIR COLLECTIVE MINDSET HELPED THEM NAVIGATE THROUGH THE UNCERTAINTIES AND CHALLENGES OF THE PANDEMIC.

DESPITE THE HARDSHIPS THEY FACED, THE LEE FAMILY DISCOVERED THE POWER OF GRATITUDE AND RESILIENCE. THEY CELEBRATED EVEN THE SMALLEST VICTORIES, FINDING JOY IN THE SIMPLE MOMENTS THEY SHARED. THEIR LOVE AND DETERMINATION BECAME THE BEDROCK

OF THEIR UNITY AND MOTIVATION TO OVERCOME OBSTACLES.

THE LEE FAMILY'S STORY IS A TESTAMENT TO THE POWER OF LOVE, DETERMINATION, AND ADAPTABILITY. THROUGH THEIR UNWAVERING COMMITMENT TO SUPPORTING ONE ANOTHER, THEY TRANSFORMED SETBACKS INTO OPPORTUNITIES FOR GROWTH. THEY DEMONSTRATED THAT A UNITED FAMILY CAN WEATHER ANY STORM AND EMERGE STRONGER ON THE OTHER SIDE.

THE LEE FAMILY'S JOURNEY SERVES AS AN INSPIRATION, REMINDING US OF THE IMPORTANCE OF LOVE, DETERMINATION, AND RESILIENCE IN NAVIGATING DIFFICULT TIMES.

THEIR STORY DEMONSTRATES THAT THROUGH UNWAVERING SUPPORT, ADAPTATION, AND AN UNYIELDING SPIRIT, FAMILIES CAN OVERCOME CHALLENGES AND CREATE A SENSE OF HOPE AND STRENGTH.

THE JOHNSON FAMILY:

THE JOHNSON FAMILY, CONSISTING OF PARENTS AND THEIR TWO CHILDREN, LIVED IN A TIGHT-KNIT COMMUNITY WHERE NEIGHBORS WERE MORE THAN JUST ACQUAINTANCES—THEY WERE LIKE EXTENDED FAMILY. WHEN THE PANDEMIC STRUCK, THE

JOHNSONS AND THEIR NEIGHBORS FOUND THEMSELVES FACING UNPRECEDENTED CHALLENGES, BUT THEIR UNITY AND SUPPORT FOR ONE ANOTHER BECAME A SOURCE OF STRENGTH.

ONE OF THE INITIAL CHALLENGES THE JOHNSONS AND THEIR NEIGHBORS ENCOUNTERED WAS THE SUDDEN DISRUPTION TO THEIR DAILY LIVES. JOBS WERE LOST, SCHOOLS CLOSED, AND SOCIAL INTERACTIONS BECAME LIMITED. HOWEVER, THEY REFUSED TO LET THESE CIRCUMSTANCES DRIVE THEM APART. INSTEAD, THEY BANDED TOGETHER, FORMING A SUPPORT NETWORK THAT WOULD PROVE ESSENTIAL IN THE MONTHS TO COME.

RECOGNIZING THE POWER OF THEIR COLLECTIVE STRENGTH, THE JOHNSON FAMILY AND THEIR NEIGHBORS ORGANIZED REGULAR VIRTUAL MEETINGS AND DISCUSSIONS. THEY SHARED INFORMATION, RESOURCES, AND EMOTIONAL SUPPORT, ENSURING THAT NO ONE FELT ALONE OR OVERWHELMED BY THE CIRCUMSTANCES. THESE GATHERINGS BECAME A LIFELINE, PROVIDING A SENSE OF COMMUNITY AND BELONGING DURING A TIME OF ISOLATION.

ONE OF THE MAJOR CHALLENGES THEY FACED WAS THE LIMITED AVAILABILITY OF ESSENTIAL SUPPLIES. WITH PANIC BUYING AND SHORTAGES, OBTAINING GROCERIES AND NECESSARY ITEMS BECAME A STRUGGLE. HOWEVER, THE JOHNSONS AND THEIR NEIGHBORS FOUND A SOLUTION BY

ESTABLISHING A COMMUNITY SUPPORT SYSTEM. THEY ORGANIZED GROUP ORDERS, SHARED DELIVERIES, AND EVEN CREATED A COMMUNITY GARDEN WHERE THEY COULD GROW FRESH PRODUCE TOGETHER. THROUGH THEIR COLLABORATION, THEY ENSURED THAT EVERYONE HAD ACCESS TO VITAL RESOURCES AND THAT NO ONE WENT WITHOUT.

ADDITIONALLY, THE JOHNSONS AND THEIR NEIGHBORS FACED THE CHALLENGE OF REMOTE LEARNING FOR THEIR CHILDREN. WITH SCHOOLS CLOSED, THEY WORKED COLLECTIVELY TO ADDRESS THE EDUCATIONAL NEEDS OF THEIR KIDS. THEY ORGANIZED STUDY GROUPS, SHARED ONLINE RESOURCES, AND TOOK TURNS PROVIDING VIRTUAL TUTORING

AND MENTORSHIP. BY POOLING THEIR KNOWLEDGE AND RESOURCES, THEY ENSURED THAT THE CHILDREN CONTINUED TO RECEIVE QUALITY EDUCATION AND SUPPORT DESPITE THE CHALLENGING CIRCUMSTANCES.

BEYOND PRACTICAL MATTERS, THE JOHNSONS AND THEIR NEIGHBORS ALSO RECOGNIZED THE IMPORTANCE OF EMOTIONAL WELL-BEING. THEY REGULARLY CHECKED IN ON ONE ANOTHER, OFFERING A LISTENING EAR AND A SHOULDER TO LEAN ON. THEY ORGANIZED VIRTUAL SOCIAL GATHERINGS, INCLUDING GAME NIGHTS, MOVIE MARATHONS, AND EVEN VIRTUAL EXERCISE SESSIONS. THEIR COMMITMENT TO NURTURING THEIR COLLECTIVE WELL-BEING CREATED A

SENSE OF CAMARADERIE AND EMOTIONAL SUPPORT WITHIN THE COMMUNITY.

THROUGH THEIR COLLECTIVE RESILIENCE AND SUPPORT FOR ONE ANOTHER, THE JOHNSON FAMILY AND THEIR NEIGHBORS DEMONSTRATED THE POWER OF UNITY IN THE FACE OF ADVERSITY. THEY EXEMPLIFIED THE NOTION THAT A STRONG COMMUNITY CAN WEATHER ANY STORM BY STANDING TOGETHER, SUPPORTING ONE ANOTHER, AND FINDING INNOVATIVE SOLUTIONS TO SHARED CHALLENGES.

THE STORY OF THE JOHNSON FAMILY AND THEIR NEIGHBORS SERVES AS A POWERFUL REMINDER THAT IN TIMES OF CRISIS, THE BONDS OF

COMMUNITY AND SOLIDARITY CAN PROVIDE STRENGTH, SUPPORT, AND RESILIENCE. THEIR COLLECTIVE DETERMINATION TO UPLIFT ONE ANOTHER, SHARE RESOURCES, AND PROVIDE EMOTIONAL SUPPORT SHOWCASES THE BEST OF HUMANITY. TOGETHER, THEY NAVIGATED THE HARDSHIPS OF THE PANDEMIC, EMERGING STRONGER AND MORE CONNECTED THAN EVER BEFORE.

STUDENTS AND

EDUCATION

THE COVID-19 PANDEMIC HAS HAD A PROFOUND AND LASTING IMPACT ON STUDENTS WORLDWIDE, UPENDING THEIR EDUCATIONAL JOURNEY AND SIGNIFICANTLY AFFECTING THEIR EMOTIONAL WELL-BEING. AS SCHOOLS SHIFTED TO REMOTE LEARNING AND PHYSICAL DISTANCING MEASURES WERE IMPLEMENTED, STUDENTS FOUND THEMSELVES FACING A MYRIAD OF CHALLENGES, LEADING TO A RANGE OF EMOTIONAL RESPONSES.

ONE OF THE MOST PREVALENT AND DEEPLY FELT EMOTIONS EXPERIENCED BY STUDENTS DURING THIS TIME WAS A SENSE OF PROFOUND ISOLATION. THE SUDDEN TRANSITION TO ONLINE CLASSES MEANT THAT STUDENTS WERE PHYSICALLY SEPARATED FROM THEIR PEERS AND TEACHERS, MISSING OUT ON THE SOCIAL INTERACTIONS AND SUPPORT SYSTEMS TYPICALLY FOUND IN SCHOOLS. THE ABSENCE OF FACE-TO-FACE CONNECTIONS, THE LOSS OF EVERYDAY SCHOOL ROUTINES, AND THE LACK OF CASUAL CONVERSATIONS IN HALLWAYS AND LUNCHROOMS LEFT MANY STUDENTS FEELING DISCONNECTED AND LONELY.

FURTHERMORE, THE DISRUPTION TO EXTRACURRICULAR ACTIVITIES, SUCH AS

SPORTS, CLUBS, AND EVENTS, FURTHER INTENSIFIED THE SENSE OF ISOLATION. THESE ACTIVITIES NOT ONLY PROVIDED OPPORTUNITIES FOR PERSONAL GROWTH AND DEVELOPMENT BUT ALSO SERVED AS OUTLETS FOR STRESS RELIEF AND SOCIAL CONNECTIONS. WITHOUT THESE OUTLETS, STUDENTS FELT A VOID IN THEIR LIVES, EXACERBATING THEIR FEELINGS OF LONELINESS AND DETACHMENT.

THE CONSTANT UNCERTAINTY SURROUNDING THE PANDEMIC ALSO FUELED ANXIETY AMONG STUDENTS. CONCERNS ABOUT THEIR OWN HEALTH AND THE HEALTH OF THEIR LOVED ONES, AS WELL AS THE FEAR OF CONTRACTING THE VIRUS, WEIGHED HEAVILY ON THEIR MINDS. THE SUDDEN CHANGES IN ACADEMIC FORMATS

AND THE CHALLENGES OF ADAPTING TO ONLINE LEARNING ADDED TO THEIR ANXIETY LEVELS. THE PRESSURE TO PERFORM WELL ACADEMICALLY UNDER THESE NEW CIRCUMSTANCES AND THE UNCERTAINTIES ABOUT THE FUTURE TOOK A TOLL ON THEIR MENTAL WELL-BEING.

ACADEMIC CHALLENGES WERE ALSO A SIGNIFICANT SOURCE OF STRESS FOR STUDENTS DURING THE PANDEMIC. THE TRANSITION TO REMOTE LEARNING PRESENTED UNIQUE OBSTACLES, SUCH AS DIFFICULTIES IN STAYING FOCUSED, MANAGING TIME EFFECTIVELY, AND ADAPTING TO NEW ONLINE PLATFORMS. THE LACK OF IN-PERSON GUIDANCE AND SUPPORT FROM TEACHERS MADE IT HARDER FOR

STUDENTS TO SEEK CLARIFICATION OR ASSISTANCE WHEN NEEDED. THIS LED TO FEELINGS OF FRUSTRATION, HELPLESSNESS, AND A DECLINE IN MOTIVATION.

ADDITIONALLY, THE DIGITAL DIVIDE FURTHER EXACERBATED THE ACADEMIC CHALLENGES. STUDENTS FROM DISADVANTAGED BACKGROUNDS OFTEN FACED BARRIERS TO ACCESSING RELIABLE INTERNET CONNECTIONS, COMPUTERS, OR OTHER NECESSARY TECHNOLOGY, PUTTING THEM AT A SIGNIFICANT DISADVANTAGE IN THEIR EDUCATIONAL PURSUITS. THIS INEQUALITY ADDED AN EXTRA LAYER OF STRESS AND FRUSTRATION FOR THOSE STUDENTS WHO STRUGGLED TO KEEP UP WITH THEIR PEERS.

THE PROLONGED NATURE OF THE PANDEMIC AND THE ONGOING UNCERTAINTIES HAVE ALSO TAKEN A TOLL ON STUDENTS' MENTAL HEALTH. THE DISRUPTION TO THEIR ROUTINES, THE LACK OF SOCIAL INTERACTION, AND THE CONSTANT BARRAGE OF PANDEMIC-RELATED NEWS HAVE CONTRIBUTED TO FEELINGS OF OVERWHELM, SADNESS, AND ANXIETY. MANY STUDENTS HAVE EXPERIENCED A SENSE OF GRIEF OVER THE LOSS OF NORMALCY, MILESTONES, AND THE TRADITIONAL SCHOOL EXPERIENCE.

IT IS CRUCIAL TO RECOGNIZE AND ADDRESS THESE EMOTIONAL STRUGGLES FACED BY STUDENTS DURING THE PANDEMIC. SCHOOLS, PARENTS, AND COMMUNITIES MUST COME TOGETHER TO PROVIDE SUPPORT SYSTEMS AND

RESOURCES TO HELP STUDENTS NAVIGATE THROUGH THESE CHALLENGING TIMES. BY FOSTERING A SENSE OF COMMUNITY, PROMOTING OPEN COMMUNICATION, AND PROVIDING ACCESS TO MENTAL HEALTH SERVICES, WE CAN HELP STUDENTS COPE WITH THEIR EMOTIONS, REGAIN A SENSE OF NORMALCY, AND THRIVE ACADEMICALLY AND EMOTIONALLY DESPITE THE ONGOING CHALLENGES POSED BY THE PANDEMIC.

IT IS ALSO IMPORTANT TO ACKNOWLEDGE THE RESILIENCE AND STRENGTH EXHIBITED BY STUDENTS DURING THESE CHALLENGING TIMES. MANY HAVE SHOWN INCREDIBLE ADAPTABILITY, CREATIVITY, AND DETERMINATION IN FINDING WAYS TO CONTINUE THEIR EDUCATION,

CONNECT WITH PEERS VIRTUALLY, AND SUPPORT ONE ANOTHER. THEIR ABILITY TO NAVIGATE THROUGH ADVERSITY SPEAKS TO THEIR CAPACITY FOR GROWTH AND RESILIENCE.

AS WE MOVE FORWARD, IT IS ESSENTIAL TO PRIORITIZE THE HOLISTIC WELL-BEING OF STUDENTS, ADDRESSING THEIR EMOTIONAL NEEDS ALONGSIDE THEIR ACADEMIC PROGRESS. BY CREATING A SUPPORTIVE AND INCLUSIVE ENVIRONMENT, OFFERING MENTAL HEALTH RESOURCES, AND PROVIDING OPPORTUNITIES FOR MEANINGFUL CONNECTION AND ENGAGEMENT, WE CAN HELP STUDENTS NOT ONLY SURVIVE

SARAH'S DETERMINATION:

SARAH, A HIGH SCHOOL STUDENT, EXEMPLIFIES UNWAVERING DETERMINATION AND RESILIENCE IN THE FACE OF CHALLENGING CIRCUMSTANCES DURING THE PANDEMIC. WHEN HER SCHOOL SHIFTED TO REMOTE LEARNING, SHE ENCOUNTERED A SIGNIFICANT OBSTACLE: SHE DIDN'T HAVE RELIABLE INTERNET ACCESS AT HOME.

RATHER THAN ALLOWING THIS SETBACK TO HINDER HER EDUCATION, SARAH TOOK MATTERS INTO HER OWN HANDS. SHE RECOGNIZED THE IMPORTANCE OF ATTENDING ONLINE CLASSES AND COMPLETING ASSIGNMENTS, AND SHE REFUSED TO LET THE LACK OF INTERNET ACCESS HOLD HER BACK. EVERY DAY, SARAH WOKE UP EARLY AND EMBARKED ON A JOURNEY TO THE NEARBY LIBRARY.

DESPITE THE ADDED EFFORT AND THE EARLY MORNINGS, SARAH WAS DETERMINED TO MAKE THE MOST OF HER EDUCATIONAL OPPORTUNITIES. SHE WALKED TO THE LIBRARY, WHERE SHE COULD ACCESS THE INTERNET AND PARTICIPATE IN HER ONLINE CLASSES. WITH A THIRST FOR KNOWLEDGE AND A COMMITMENT TO HER STUDIES, SARAH DEDICATED HERSELF TO LEARNING IN A WAY THAT WENT ABOVE AND BEYOND WHAT WAS EXPECTED.

SARAH'S DETERMINATION SERVES AS A POWERFUL REMINDER OF THE LENGTHS STUDENTS ARE WILLING TO GO TO OVERCOME

OBSTACLES. HER STORY SHOWCASES THE RESILIENCE AND ADAPTABILITY OF YOUNG INDIVIDUALS WHO REFUSE TO LET CIRCUMSTANCES DICTATE THEIR EDUCATIONAL PURSUITS. SARAH'S UNWAVERING COMMITMENT TO ATTENDING CLASSES AND COMPLETING ASSIGNMENTS DESPITE THE LACK OF INTERNET ACCESS DEMONSTRATES HER DEEP APPRECIATION FOR EDUCATION AND HER UNYIELDING DRIVE TO SUCCEED.

SARAH'S STORY ALSO HIGHLIGHTS THE IMPORTANCE OF RECOGNIZING AND ADDRESSING THE DIGITAL DIVIDE THAT EXISTS AMONG STUDENTS, AS IT CAN SIGNIFICANTLY IMPACT THEIR ABILITY TO ACCESS EDUCATIONAL RESOURCES. HER DETERMINATION SERVES AS A CALL TO ACTION TO ENSURE THAT ALL STUDENTS HAVE EQUITABLE ACCESS TO THE TOOLS AND RESOURCES NECESSARY TO PURSUE THEIR EDUCATION, REGARDLESS OF THEIR CIRCUMSTANCES.

OVERALL, SARAH'S DETERMINATION IS AN INSPIRING EXAMPLE OF HOW STUDENTS CAN OVERCOME CHALLENGES WITH GRIT AND PERSEVERANCE. HER STORY SERVES AS A SOURCE OF MOTIVATION AND ENCOURAGEMENT FOR OTHERS WHO MAY BE FACING SIMILAR OBSTACLES, SHOWING THAT WITH DETERMINATION, RESOURCEFULNESS, AND A THIRST FOR KNOWLEDGE, ONE CAN TRIUMPH OVER ADVERSITY AND ACHIEVE ACADEMIC SUCCESS.

ALEX'S ENTREPRENEURIAL SPIRIT:

ALEX, A COLLEGE STUDENT, DEMONSTRATED REMARKABLE ENTREPRENEURIAL SPIRIT AND ADAPTABILITY DURING THE PANDEMIC. WHEN HE LOST HIS PART-TIME JOB DUE TO THE ECONOMIC IMPACT OF THE CRISIS, HE REFUSED TO LET IT DETER HIM FROM SUPPORTING HIMSELF AND CONTINUING HIS EDUCATION.

INSTEAD OF SUCCUMBING TO THE SETBACK, ALEX TAPPED INTO HIS CREATIVITY AND RESOURCEFULNESS TO FIND A SOLUTION. HE DECIDED TO LEVERAGE HIS SKILLS AND INTERESTS TO START A SMALL ONLINE BUSINESS. DRAWING ON HIS PASSION FOR CRAFTING AND CREATING HANDMADE ITEMS, ALEX BEGAN DESIGNING AND PRODUCING UNIQUE CRAFTS FROM THE COMFORT OF HIS HOME.

WITH A KEEN EYE FOR AESTHETICS AND ATTENTION TO DETAIL, ALEX CRAFTED A RANGE OF PRODUCTS, INCLUDING JEWELRY, ARTWORK, AND CUSTOMIZED ACCESSORIES. HE SET UP AN ONLINE STORE TO SHOWCASE AND SELL HIS CREATIONS, REACHING CUSTOMERS FAR BEYOND HIS IMMEDIATE COMMUNITY.

THROUGH HIS ENTREPRENEURIAL VENTURE, ALEX NOT ONLY GENERATED INCOME BUT ALSO GAINED VALUABLE REAL-WORLD EXPERIENCE IN MARKETING, CUSTOMER RELATIONS, AND FINANCIAL MANAGEMENT. HE LEARNED HOW TO NAVIGATE THE INTRICACIES OF RUNNING A BUSINESS, FROM SOURCING MATERIALS TO

MANAGING INVENTORY AND FULFILLING ORDERS.

ALEX'S ENTREPRENEURIAL SPIRIT IS AN INSPIRATION TO OTHER STUDENTS, SHOWCASING THE POWER OF ADAPTABILITY AND EMBRACING OPPORTUNITIES AMIDST ADVERSITY. RATHER THAN PASSIVELY WAITING FOR CIRCUMSTANCES TO IMPROVE, HE TOOK PROACTIVE STEPS TO CREATE HIS OWN PATH AND PURSUE HIS AMBITIONS.

FURTHERMORE, ALEX'S ENTREPRENEURIAL ENDEAVOR SERVED AS A TESTAMENT TO THE IMPORTANCE OF DIVERSIFYING INCOME STREAMS AND EXPLORING ALTERNATIVE AVENUES FOR FINANCIAL STABILITY. BY HARNESSING HIS CREATIVITY AND LEVERAGING HIS SKILLS, HE FOUND A WAY TO NOT ONLY SUPPORT HIMSELF BUT ALSO CONTINUE HIS EDUCATION.

ALEX'S STORY ALSO UNDERSCORES THE RESILIENCE AND DETERMINATION OF YOUNG INDIVIDUALS WHO REFUSE TO LET SETBACKS

DEFINE THEIR FUTURE. HIS ENTREPRENEURIAL JOURNEY EXEMPLIFIES THE SPIRIT OF INNOVATION, ADAPTABILITY, AND THE ABILITY TO TURN CHALLENGES INTO OPPORTUNITIES.

IN CONCLUSION, ALEX'S ENTREPRENEURIAL SPIRIT DURING THE PANDEMIC DEMONSTRATES HOW STUDENTS CAN HARNESS THEIR TALENTS, PURSUE THEIR PASSIONS, AND OVERCOME FINANCIAL OBSTACLES THROUGH CREATIVE AND ENTREPRENEURIAL ENDEAVORS. HIS STORY SERVES AS A REMINDER THAT WITH A THIRST FOR KNOWLEDGE, RESOURCEFULNESS, AND THE WILLINGNESS TO TAKE CALCULATED RISKS, STUDENTS CAN NOT ONLY SURVIVE BUT THRIVE IN CHALLENGING TIMES.

MAYA'S GLOBAL CONNECTIONS

MAYA, A MIDDLE SCHOOL STUDENT, EXEMPLIFIED A REMARKABLE SENSE OF CURIOSITY, OPEN-MINDEDNESS, AND ADAPTABILITY DURING THE PANDEMIC. DESPITE

THE PHYSICAL DISTANCE IMPOSED BY REMOTE
LEARNING AND THE LIMITATIONS ON TRAVEL
AND IN-PERSON INTERACTIONS, MAYA
DISCOVERED NEW WAYS TO CONNECT WITH
PEERS FROM AROUND THE WORLD, EXPANDING
HER HORIZONS AND FOSTERING GLOBAL
CONNECTIONS.

RECOGNIZING THE IMPORTANCE OF CULTURAL
EXCHANGE AND UNDERSTANDING, MAYA
ACTIVELY SOUGHT OUT VIRTUAL
OPPORTUNITIES TO ENGAGE WITH STUDENTS
FROM DIFFERENT COUNTRIES AND
BACKGROUNDS. SHE PARTICIPATED IN ONLINE
INTERNATIONAL COLLABORATIONS, LANGUAGE
EXCHANGE PROGRAMS, AND VIRTUAL
CULTURAL EVENTS. THROUGH THESE
PLATFORMS, MAYA HAD THE CHANCE TO
CONNECT WITH STUDENTS HER AGE WHO
SHARED DIFFERENT LANGUAGES, TRADITIONS,
AND PERSPECTIVES.

THROUGH THESE VIRTUAL INTERACTIONS,
MAYA DEVELOPED MEANINGFUL FRIENDSHIPS
AND GAINED A DEEPER UNDERSTANDING OF

DIVERSE CULTURES AND WORLDVIEWS. SHE ENGAGED IN CONVERSATIONS, SHARED EXPERIENCES, AND EXCHANGED IDEAS, BROADENING HER PERSPECTIVE AND CHALLENGING HER ASSUMPTIONS. MAYA'S COMMITMENT TO GLOBAL CONNECTIONS SHOWCASED HER EAGERNESS TO LEARN FROM OTHERS AND HER APPRECIATION FOR THE RICHNESS OF HUMAN DIVERSITY.

DESPITE THE CHALLENGES OF PHYSICAL SEPARATION AND LIMITED TRAVEL, MAYA'S VIRTUAL CONNECTIONS TRANSCENDED BORDERS AND SERVED AS A REMINDER OF THE POWER OF TECHNOLOGY IN FOSTERING GLOBAL UNDERSTANDING AND EMPATHY. THROUGH HER ACTIVE PARTICIPATION IN THESE VIRTUAL PLATFORMS, MAYA NOT ONLY EXPANDED HER KNOWLEDGE BUT ALSO CONTRIBUTED TO BUILDING BRIDGES OF FRIENDSHIP AND COOPERATION ACROSS CONTINENTS.

MAYA'S STORY SERVES AS AN INSPIRATION TO OTHER STUDENTS, HIGHLIGHTING THE IMPORTANCE OF EMBRACING OPPORTUNITIES

FOR CULTURAL EXCHANGE AND SEEKING CONNECTIONS BEYOND ONE'S IMMEDIATE SURROUNDINGS. HER CURIOSITY, OPEN-MINDEDNESS, AND ADAPTABILITY ALLOWED HER TO OVERCOME PHYSICAL BARRIERS AND ENGAGE IN MEANINGFUL VIRTUAL CONNECTIONS WITH STUDENTS FROM DIVERSE BACKGROUNDS.

BY EMBRACING VIRTUAL PLATFORMS AND ACTIVELY PARTICIPATING IN INTERNATIONAL COLLABORATIONS, MAYA DEMONSTRATED THAT EVEN DURING CHALLENGING TIMES, THERE ARE STILL AVENUES FOR LEARNING, CONNECTION, AND GLOBAL UNDERSTANDING. HER STORY ENCOURAGES OTHER STUDENTS TO EXPLORE VIRTUAL OPPORTUNITIES, CHALLENGE THEIR PRECONCEPTIONS, AND ENGAGE IN MEANINGFUL CONVERSATIONS WITH PEERS FROM DIFFERENT CULTURES AND PERSPECTIVES.

IN CONCLUSION, MAYA'S PURSUIT OF GLOBAL CONNECTIONS AMIDST THE PANDEMIC EXEMPLIFIES THE POWER OF CURIOSITY,

OPEN-MINDEDNESS, AND ADAPTABILITY. HER STORY REMINDS US THAT DESPITE PHYSICAL DISTANCE, WE CAN FOSTER CONNECTIONS, LEARN FROM OTHERS, AND BUILD BRIDGES OF UNDERSTANDING AND FRIENDSHIP THAT TRANSCEND BORDERS. MAYA'S DEDICATION TO GLOBAL CONNECTIONS SERVES AS AN INSPIRATION FOR STUDENTS TO ACTIVELY SEEK OPPORTUNITIES FOR CULTURAL EXCHANGE AND BROADEN THEIR HORIZONS, EVEN IN CHALLENGING TIMES.

DAVID'S INNOVATIVE SOLUTIONS:

DAVID, A UNIVERSITY STUDENT STUDYING ENGINEERING, SHOWCASED REMARKABLE CREATIVITY, PROBLEM-SOLVING SKILLS, AND ADAPTABILITY DURING THE PANDEMIC. FACED WITH THE CHALLENGES OF HANDS-ON PROJECTS THAT WERE TRADITIONALLY CONDUCTED IN LABS, HE EMBRACED THE OPPORTUNITY TO FIND INNOVATIVE SOLUTIONS AND BRIDGE THE GAP BETWEEN VIRTUAL LEARNING AND PRACTICAL APPLICATION.

RECOGNIZING THE LIMITATIONS IMPOSED BY REMOTE LEARNING, DAVID TOOK IT UPON HIMSELF TO DEVELOP A VIRTUAL LAB PLATFORM. THIS PLATFORM ALLOWED STUDENTS TO SIMULATE EXPERIMENTS AND ENGAGE IN COLLABORATIVE LEARNING EXPERIENCES REMOTELY. THROUGH HIS TECHNICAL SKILLS AND INGENUITY, DAVID CREATED AN IMMERSIVE VIRTUAL ENVIRONMENT THAT REPLICATED THE HANDS-ON ASPECTS OF THEIR COURSEWORK.

BY DESIGNING THE VIRTUAL LAB PLATFORM, DAVID NOT ONLY ADDRESSED THE ACADEMIC CHALLENGES POSED BY THE PANDEMIC BUT ALSO PROVIDED HIS PEERS WITH AN ALTERNATIVE MEANS OF PRACTICAL LEARNING. STUDENTS WERE ABLE TO CONDUCT EXPERIMENTS, ANALYZE DATA, AND COLLABORATE WITH THEIR CLASSMATES, ALL WITHIN THE VIRTUAL LAB ENVIRONMENT DAVID HAD CREATED.

DAVID'S INNOVATIVE SOLUTION DEMONSTRATED HIS ABILITY TO THINK

OUTSIDE THE BOX AND ADAPT TO CHANGING CIRCUMSTANCES. HIS PROJECT NOT ONLY BENEFITED HIMSELF BUT ALSO HAD A POSITIVE IMPACT ON HIS PEERS, ENABLING THEM TO CONTINUE THEIR ACADEMIC PROGRESS DESPITE THE LIMITATIONS IMPOSED BY REMOTE LEARNING.

MOREOVER, DAVID'S INITIATIVE SHOWCASED THE POTENTIAL OF TECHNOLOGY IN ENHANCING THE EDUCATIONAL EXPERIENCE. HIS VIRTUAL LAB PLATFORM NOT ONLY PROVIDED A WORKAROUND DURING THE PANDEMIC BUT ALSO OPENED UP POSSIBILITIES FOR REMOTE LEARNING EVEN BEYOND THE IMMEDIATE CRISIS. THE PLATFORM COULD BE FURTHER DEVELOPED AND EXPANDED TO REACH STUDENTS IN REMOTE AREAS, OFFERING THEM ACCESS TO PRACTICAL LEARNING EXPERIENCES THAT MIGHT OTHERWISE BE UNAVAILABLE.

DAVID'S STORY SERVES AS AN INSPIRATION TO OTHER STUDENTS, HIGHLIGHTING THE IMPORTANCE OF INNOVATIVE THINKING,

PROBLEM-SOLVING SKILLS, AND THE ABILITY TO ADAPT TO CHANGING CIRCUMSTANCES. HIS DEDICATION TO FINDING A SOLUTION AND HIS WILLINGNESS TO SHARE IT WITH HIS PEERS EXEMPLIFY THE SPIRIT OF COLLABORATION AND SUPPORT WITHIN THE ACADEMIC COMMUNITY.

IN CONCLUSION, DAVID'S INNOVATIVE SOLUTION IN CREATING A VIRTUAL LAB PLATFORM DEMONSTRATES THE POWER OF CREATIVITY, PROBLEM-SOLVING, AND ADAPTABILITY IN OVERCOMING CHALLENGES. HIS STORY EMPHASIZES THE POTENTIAL OF TECHNOLOGY TO BRIDGE GAPS IN EDUCATION AND PROVIDE PRACTICAL LEARNING EXPERIENCES, EVEN IN TIMES OF CRISIS. DAVID'S INITIATIVE SERVES AS A REMINDER THAT WITH THE RIGHT MINDSET AND A WILLINGNESS TO EXPLORE NEW POSSIBILITIES, STUDENTS CAN FIND INNOVATIVE SOLUTIONS TO CONTINUE THEIR EDUCATIONAL JOURNEY AND INSPIRE OTHERS ALONG THE WAY.

MIA'S COMMITMENT TO SERVICE:

MIA, A HIGH SCHOOL STUDENT, DEMONSTRATED EXCEPTIONAL COMPASSION, LEADERSHIP, AND A COMMITMENT TO SERVING HER COMMUNITY DURING THE CHALLENGING TIMES OF THE PANDEMIC. RECOGNIZING THE INCREASED NEED FOR SUPPORT, PARTICULARLY AMONG YOUNGER STUDENTS STRUGGLING WITH REMOTE LEARNING, MIA TOOK IT UPON HERSELF TO INITIATE A VOLUNTEER GROUP DEDICATED TO PROVIDING VIRTUAL TUTORING AND MENTORING.

DRIVEN BY HER EMPATHY AND UNDERSTANDING OF THE DIFFICULTIES FACED BY YOUNGER STUDENTS, MIA GATHERED A GROUP OF LIKE-MINDED PEERS WHO SHARED HER PASSION FOR HELPING OTHERS. TOGETHER, THEY FORMED A SUPPORTIVE NETWORK OF VOLUNTEERS WHO DEDICATED THEIR TIME AND EXPERTISE TO ASSIST YOUNGER STUDENTS IN NAVIGATING THE CHALLENGES OF REMOTE LEARNING.

MIA'S COMMITMENT TO SERVICE WAS EVIDENT IN HER DEDICATION TO ORGANIZING AND

COORDINATING THE ACTIVITIES OF THE VOLUNTEER GROUP. SHE MATCHED TUTORS WITH STUDENTS, FACILITATED VIRTUAL TUTORING SESSIONS, AND ENSURED ONGOING COMMUNICATION AND SUPPORT BETWEEN THE VOLUNTEERS AND THE STUDENTS THEY WERE HELPING.

THROUGH MIA'S LEADERSHIP, THE VOLUNTEER GROUP BECAME A SOURCE OF ENCOURAGEMENT, ACADEMIC ASSISTANCE, AND EMOTIONAL SUPPORT FOR THE YOUNGER STUDENTS. BY PROVIDING ONE-ON-ONE TUTORING, MENTORING, AND A LISTENING EAR, THEY HELPED ALLEVIATE THE ISOLATION, ANXIETY, AND ACADEMIC CHALLENGES THAT MANY STUDENTS WERE FACING DURING THE PANDEMIC.

MIA'S INITIATIVE AND COMMITMENT TO SERVICE HAD A PROFOUND IMPACT ON THE LIVES OF THE STUDENTS SHE AND HER TEAM SUPPORTED. BEYOND ACADEMIC IMPROVEMENT, THE RELATIONSHIPS BUILT THROUGH THIS PROGRAM FOSTERED A SENSE OF BELONGING,

MOTIVATION, AND CONFIDENCE AMONG THE YOUNGER STUDENTS, EMPOWERING THEM TO PERSEVERE THROUGH THE DIFFICULTIES THEY WERE FACING.

MIA'S STORY IS AN INSPIRATION TO OTHER STUDENTS, DEMONSTRATING THE POWER OF COMPASSION, LEADERSHIP, AND SERVICE. HER DEDICATION TO SUPPORTING HER COMMUNITY DURING A TIME OF CRISIS EXEMPLIFIES THE POSITIVE IMPACT THAT YOUNG INDIVIDUALS CAN HAVE WHEN THEY STEP UP AND TAKE ACTION.

FURTHERMORE, MIA'S COMMITMENT TO SERVICE HIGHLIGHTS THE IMPORTANCE OF FOSTERING A CULTURE OF EMPATHY, SUPPORT, AND GIVING BACK WITHIN EDUCATIONAL COMMUNITIES. HER VOLUNTEER GROUP SERVED AS A TESTAMENT TO THE RESILIENCE AND KINDNESS THAT CAN FLOURISH EVEN IN CHALLENGING TIMES.

IN CONCLUSION, MIA'S COMMITMENT TO SERVICE EXEMPLIFIES THE PROFOUND IMPACT

THAT INDIVIDUALS CAN HAVE ON THEIR COMMUNITIES BY EXTENDING A HELPING HAND TO THOSE IN NEED. HER STORY SERVES AS A REMINDER OF THE IMPORTANCE OF COMPASSION, LEADERSHIP, AND THE TRANSFORMATIVE POWER OF SERVICE, INSPIRING OTHERS TO MAKE A DIFFERENCE IN THEIR OWN COMMUNITIES AND SUPPORT ONE ANOTHER THROUGH ACTS OF KINDNESS AND SUPPORT.

THESE INSPIRING STORIES DEMONSTRATE THE RESILIENCE, ADAPTABILITY, AND THIRST FOR KNOWLEDGE EXHIBITED BY STUDENTS DURING CHALLENGING TIMES. THEIR STORIES REMIND US THAT EVEN IN THE FACE OF ADVERSITY, YOUNG INDIVIDUALS HAVE THE CAPACITY TO RISE ABOVE OBSTACLES, PURSUE THEIR EDUCATIONAL GOALS, AND MAKE A DIFFERENCE IN THEIR COMMUNITIES. THEIR DETERMINATION AND INNOVATION SERVE AS INSPIRATION FOR OTHERS, SHOWING THAT

LEARNING AND PERSONAL GROWTH CAN THRIVE UNDER ANY CIRCUMSTANCES.

BUSINESS AND ECONOMIC CHALLENGES

THE EMOTIONAL IMPACT OF JOB LOSS, FINANCIAL INSTABILITY, AND THE FEAR OF BUSINESS CLOSURE IS PROFOUND AND FAR-REACHING. IT GOES BEYOND THE IMMEDIATE CONCERNS OF FINANCES AND ECONOMIC STABILITY, AFFECTING INDIVIDUALS

AND FAMILIES ON A DEEPLY PERSONAL AND EMOTIONAL LEVEL.

JOB LOSS CAN BRING ABOUT A SENSE OF SHOCK, DISBELIEF, AND A LOSS OF IDENTITY. SUDDENLY FINDING ONESELF UNEMPLOYED CAN LEAD TO FEELINGS OF INADEQUACY, SELF-DOUBT, AND A LOSS OF PURPOSE. IT CAN BE A DEVASTATING BLOW TO ONE'S SELF-ESTEEM AND MENTAL WELL-BEING, AS INDIVIDUALS GRAPPLE WITH THE UNCERTAINTY OF THEIR FUTURE AND THEIR ABILITY TO PROVIDE FOR THEMSELVES AND THEIR LOVED ONES.

FINANCIAL INSTABILITY ADDS ANOTHER LAYER OF STRESS AND ANXIETY. THE INABILITY TO MEET FINANCIAL OBLIGATIONS, SUCH AS BILLS, MORTGAGE OR RENT PAYMENTS, AND BASIC NECESSITIES, CAN CAUSE A CONSTANT STATE OF WORRY AND FEAR. THE FEAR OF NOT BEING ABLE TO MAKE ENDS MEET AND SLIPPING INTO POVERTY CAN BE OVERWHELMING, LEADING TO FEELINGS OF HELPLESSNESS, FRUSTRATION, AND EVEN SHAME.

FOR BUSINESS OWNERS, THE FEAR OF BUSINESS CLOSURE CARRIES A HEAVY EMOTIONAL BURDEN. MANY ENTREPRENEURS POUR THEIR HEARTS AND SOULS INTO BUILDING THEIR BUSINESSES, AND THE PROSPECT OF SEEING THEIR DREAMS SHATTERED CAN BE DEVASTATING. THE STRESS AND PRESSURE OF MAKING DIFFICULT DECISIONS, SUCH AS LAYING OFF EMPLOYEES OR SHUTTING DOWN OPERATIONS, WEIGH HEAVILY ON THEIR SHOULDERS. THE EMOTIONAL TOLL OF LETTING GO OF EMPLOYEES WHO HAVE BECOME LIKE FAMILY AND FACING THE UNCERTAINTY OF THE FUTURE CAN BE HEART-WRENCHING.

THESE EMOTIONAL IMPACTS EXTEND BEYOND THE INDIVIDUALS DIRECTLY AFFECTED TO THEIR FAMILIES AND LOVED ONES. FINANCIAL STRAIN CAN STRAIN RELATIONSHIPS, CAUSING TENSION AND ARGUMENTS AS THE PRESSURE MOUNTS. THE EMOTIONAL TOLL OF WITNESSING A LOVED ONE'S STRUGGLE CAN LEAD TO FEELINGS OF HELPLESSNESS AND CONCERN.

THE FEAR OF JOB LOSS AND FINANCIAL INSTABILITY ALSO TAKES A TOLL ON MENTAL HEALTH. ANXIETY, DEPRESSION, AND OTHER MENTAL HEALTH ISSUES CAN ARISE OR WORSEN AS INDIVIDUALS GRAPPLE WITH THE UNCERTAINTY AND STRESS OF THEIR SITUATION. THE CONSTANT WORRY AND SLEEPLESS NIGHTS CAN LEAD TO A SENSE OF HOPELESSNESS AND DESPAIR.

IT IS IMPORTANT TO RECOGNIZE AND ADDRESS THE EMOTIONAL IMPACT OF JOB LOSS, FINANCIAL INSTABILITY, AND THE FEAR OF BUSINESS CLOSURE. PROVIDING EMOTIONAL SUPPORT, COUNSELING SERVICES, AND RESOURCES FOR INDIVIDUALS AND FAMILIES CAN HELP THEM NAVIGATE THE CHALLENGING EMOTIONAL LANDSCAPE. CREATING A SUPPORTIVE ENVIRONMENT WHERE INDIVIDUALS FEEL HEARD, UNDERSTOOD, AND EMPOWERED CAN GO A LONG WAY IN HELPING THEM COPE WITH THESE DIFFICULT CIRCUMSTANCES AND REBUILD THEIR LIVES.

SARAH'S FOOD PANTRY:

SARAH, A RESTAURANT OWNER, FOUND HERSELF FACING A SIGNIFICANT DECLINE IN BUSINESS AND A POTENTIAL CLOSURE DUE TO THE IMPACT OF THE PANDEMIC. HOWEVER, INSTEAD OF SUCCUMBING TO THE CHALLENGES, SHE EMBRACED A SPIRIT OF COURAGE, INNOVATION, AND A DEEP SENSE OF COMMUNITY.

REALIZING THAT MANY INDIVIDUALS AND FAMILIES WERE STRUGGLING WITH FOOD INSECURITY DURING THESE DIFFICULT TIMES, SARAH TRANSFORMED HER RESTAURANT INTO A COMMUNITY FOOD PANTRY. SHE RECOGNIZED THAT HER ESTABLISHMENT HAD THE NECESSARY INFRASTRUCTURE AND RESOURCES TO HELP ADDRESS THE PRESSING NEEDS OF THE COMMUNITY.

WITH THE SUPPORT OF HER STAFF AND A NETWORK OF VOLUNTEERS, SARAH BEGAN

COLLECTING AND DISTRIBUTING FOOD TO THOSE IN NEED. LOCAL BUSINESSES, FARMERS, AND COMMUNITY MEMBERS CAME TOGETHER, DONATING SURPLUS PRODUCE, NON-PERISHABLE ITEMS, AND MONETARY CONTRIBUTIONS TO SUPPORT SARAH'S INITIATIVE.

SARAH'S FOOD PANTRY QUICKLY BECAME A BEACON OF HOPE AND A LIFELINE FOR MANY INDIVIDUALS AND FAMILIES WHO WERE FACING FINANCIAL HARDSHIP AND STRUGGLING TO PUT FOOD ON THEIR TABLES. BY OFFERING FREE MEALS, GROCERIES, AND ESSENTIAL SUPPLIES, SHE NOT ONLY ALLEVIATED HUNGER BUT ALSO PROVIDED A SENSE OF COMFORT AND SUPPORT TO THOSE IN NEED.

HER INNOVATION AND ADAPTABILITY WERE CRUCIAL IN TRANSFORMING HER RESTAURANT INTO A FOOD DISTRIBUTION CENTER. SARAH IMPLEMENTED SAFETY PROTOCOLS TO ENSURE THE WELL-BEING OF HER STAFF AND VOLUNTEERS, WHILE ALSO MAINTAINING THE

HIGHEST STANDARDS OF FOOD HYGIENE AND QUALITY.

SARAH'S ACT OF CONVERTING HER STRUGGLING RESTAURANT INTO A COMMUNITY FOOD PANTRY NOT ONLY ADDRESSED AN IMMEDIATE NEED BUT ALSO FOSTERED A DEEP SENSE OF TOGETHERNESS AND SOLIDARITY WITHIN THE COMMUNITY. PEOPLE FROM ALL WALKS OF LIFE CAME FORWARD TO OFFER THEIR SUPPORT, WHETHER THROUGH DONATIONS, VOLUNTEER WORK, OR SPREADING THE WORD ABOUT SARAH'S INITIATIVE.

THE IMPACT OF SARAH'S FOOD PANTRY EXTENDED FAR BEYOND PROVIDING MEALS. IT BROUGHT PEOPLE TOGETHER, BRIDGING DIVIDES AND REMINDING THE COMMUNITY OF THE POWER OF COMPASSION, GENEROSITY, AND COLLECTIVE ACTION. SARAH'S UNWAVERING COMMITMENT TO SUPPORTING OTHERS IN THE FACE OF ADVERSITY INSPIRED OTHERS TO FOLLOW SUIT AND CONTRIBUTE IN WHATEVER WAY THEY COULD.

THROUGH HER COURAGE, INNOVATION, AND DEDICATION TO SERVING HER COMMUNITY, SARAH DEMONSTRATED THE IMMENSE CAPACITY FOR INDIVIDUALS TO MAKE A DIFFERENCE, EVEN IN THE MIDST OF CHALLENGING CIRCUMSTANCES. HER STORY SERVES AS A POWERFUL REMINDER THAT WHEN WE COME TOGETHER WITH A SHARED PURPOSE AND A COMMITMENT TO HELPING OTHERS, WE CAN CREATE TRANSFORMATIVE CHANGE AND SUPPORT THOSE MOST IN NEED.

SARAH'S FOOD PANTRY BECAME A SYMBOL OF RESILIENCE AND UNITY, HIGHLIGHTING THE STRENGTH OF THE HUMAN SPIRIT AND THE REMARKABLE ABILITY OF INDIVIDUALS TO ADAPT, INNOVATE, AND COME TOGETHER TO UPLIFT THEIR COMMUNITIES IN TIMES OF CRISIS.

CARLOS' ONLINE FITNESS CLASSES:

CARLOS, A FITNESS INSTRUCTOR, DISPLAYED REMARKABLE ADAPTABILITY AND A STRONG SENSE OF COMMUNITY DURING THE CHALLENGING TIMES BROUGHT ABOUT BY THE PANDEMIC. WHEN GYMS AND FITNESS CENTERS HAD TO CLOSE THEIR DOORS DUE TO SAFETY CONCERNS, CARLOS QUICKLY PIVOTED HIS APPROACH AND EMBRACED THE VIRTUAL REALM TO CONTINUE SERVING HIS CLIENTS AND SUPPORTING THEIR FITNESS JOURNEYS.

RECOGNIZING THE IMPORTANCE OF PHYSICAL AND MENTAL WELL-BEING, CARLOS DECIDED TO OFFER ONLINE FITNESS CLASSES AS AN ALTERNATIVE TO IN-PERSON WORKOUTS. WITH THE HELP OF TECHNOLOGY AND VIDEO CONFERENCING PLATFORMS, HE CREATED A

VIRTUAL FITNESS COMMUNITY WHERE INDIVIDUALS COULD JOIN HIS CLASSES FROM THE COMFORT OF THEIR OWN HOMES.

CARLOS'S ONLINE FITNESS CLASSES PROVIDED A LIFELINE FOR THOSE SEEKING TO MAINTAIN THEIR FITNESS ROUTINES AND PRIORITIZE THEIR HEALTH DURING THE LOCKDOWN PERIOD. BY LEVERAGING HIS EXPERTISE AND PASSION FOR FITNESS, HE INSPIRED AND MOTIVATED HIS CLIENTS TO STAY ACTIVE, EVEN IN THE FACE OF CHALLENGES AND LIMITATIONS.

THROUGH HIS INNOVATIVE APPROACH, CARLOS NOT ONLY BROUGHT HIS FITNESS EXPERTISE TO THE VIRTUAL SPACE BUT ALSO FOSTERED A SENSE OF CONNECTION AND COMMUNITY

AMONG HIS CLIENTS. DESPITE PHYSICAL DISTANCING MEASURES, PARTICIPANTS COULD INTERACT WITH ONE ANOTHER, SHARE THEIR PROGRESS, AND PROVIDE MUTUAL SUPPORT THROUGH ONLINE CHAT FEATURES AND SOCIAL MEDIA GROUPS.

CARLOS'S ONLINE FITNESS CLASSES CATERED TO A WIDE RANGE OF FITNESS LEVELS AND INTERESTS, ENSURING THAT EVERYONE HAD THE OPPORTUNITY TO PARTICIPATE AND BENEFIT FROM HIS EXPERTISE. HE OFFERED A VARIETY OF WORKOUTS, INCLUDING CARDIO, STRENGTH TRAINING, YOGA, AND MORE, ACCOMMODATING DIFFERENT PREFERENCES AND HELPING INDIVIDUALS MAINTAIN A WELL-ROUNDED FITNESS ROUTINE FROM HOME.

MOREOVER, CARLOS'S VIRTUAL FITNESS COMMUNITY SERVED AS A PLATFORM FOR INDIVIDUALS TO COME TOGETHER, SHARE THEIR STRUGGLES AND TRIUMPHS, AND OFFER WORDS OF ENCOURAGEMENT. PARTICIPANTS FOUND SOLACE IN KNOWING THEY WERE NOT ALONE IN THEIR FITNESS JOURNEYS AND THAT THEY HAD A SUPPORT SYSTEM OF LIKE-MINDED INDIVIDUALS FACING SIMILAR CHALLENGES.

CARLOS'S COMMITMENT TO HIS CLIENTS' WELL-BEING EXTENDED BEYOND THE VIRTUAL WORKOUTS. HE PROVIDED GUIDANCE ON NUTRITION, MENTAL HEALTH, AND OVERALL LIFESTYLE TIPS TO HELP HIS CLIENTS NAVIGATE THE UNIQUE CIRCUMSTANCES OF THE PANDEMIC. HIS HOLISTIC APPROACH ENSURED

THAT INDIVIDUALS RECEIVED COMPREHENSIVE SUPPORT TO MAINTAIN THEIR OVERALL WELL-BEING.

BY ADAPTING TO THE NEW NORMAL AND EMBRACING TECHNOLOGY, CARLOS DEMONSTRATED RESILIENCE, INNOVATION, AND A GENUINE CARE FOR THE INDIVIDUALS HE SERVED. HIS ONLINE FITNESS CLASSES BECAME A SOURCE OF MOTIVATION, INSPIRATION, AND A REMINDER OF THE IMPORTANCE OF PRIORITIZING HEALTH AND STAYING CONNECTED, EVEN DURING CHALLENGING TIMES.

CARLOS'S STORY SERVES AS AN INSPIRATION FOR OTHER FITNESS PROFESSIONALS AND

INDIVIDUALS SEEKING TO STAY ACTIVE AND CONNECTED IN A VIRTUAL WORLD. IT SHOWCASES THE POWER OF ADAPTATION, COMMUNITY BUILDING, AND LEVERAGING TECHNOLOGY TO CONTINUE SUPPORTING AND UPLIFTING OTHERS, NO MATTER THE CIRCUMSTANCES.

MARIA'S SEWING INITIATIVE:

MARIA, A TALENTED SEAMSTRESS, EXHIBITED TREMENDOUS COMPASSION AND RESOURCEFULNESS DURING THE COVID-19 PANDEMIC THROUGH HER SEWING INITIATIVE. RECOGNIZING THE URGENT NEED FOR

PERSONAL PROTECTIVE EQUIPMENT (PPE) AS THE VIRUS SPREAD RAPIDLY, MARIA TOOK IT UPON HERSELF TO CONTRIBUTE TO THE SOLUTION AND SUPPORT HER COMMUNITY.

WITH HER SEWING SKILLS AND A HEART FULL OF EMPATHY, MARIA SHIFTED HER FOCUS FROM CREATING FASHIONABLE GARMENTS TO SEWING FACE MASKS. SHE UNDERSTOOD THAT MASKS WERE CRUCIAL IN PREVENTING THE TRANSMISSION OF THE VIRUS AND PROTECTING INDIVIDUALS FROM INFECTION. DETERMINED TO MAKE A DIFFERENCE, MARIA EMBARKED ON A MISSION TO PROVIDE FREE MASKS TO ESSENTIAL WORKERS AND VULNERABLE POPULATIONS.

MARIA'S SEWING INITIATIVE QUICKLY GAINED MOMENTUM AS SHE RALLIED FELLOW SEAMSTRESSES, FRIENDS, AND FAMILY MEMBERS TO JOIN HER CAUSE. TOGETHER, THEY FORMED A NETWORK OF DEDICATED VOLUNTEERS, UTILIZING THEIR SEWING MACHINES, FABRIC, AND TIME TO PRODUCE A SUBSTANTIAL NUMBER OF MASKS.

IN ADDITION TO SEWING MASKS, MARIA ACTIVELY SOUGHT OUT PARTNERSHIPS WITH LOCAL BUSINESSES, COMMUNITY ORGANIZATIONS, AND HEALTHCARE FACILITIES. SHE COLLABORATED WITH THESE ENTITIES TO DISTRIBUTE THE MASKS TO THOSE IN NEED, ENSURING THEY REACHED THE HANDS OF ESSENTIAL WORKERS, UNDERSERVED

COMMUNITIES, AND INDIVIDUALS WHO LACKED ACCESS TO PROPER PROTECTION.

MARIA'S SEWING INITIATIVE WENT BEYOND THE ACT OF CREATING AND DISTRIBUTING MASKS. IT SERVED AS A SYMBOL OF HOPE, RESILIENCE, AND UNITY WITHIN HER COMMUNITY. PEOPLE FROM ALL WALKS OF LIFE CAME FORWARD TO SUPPORT HER CAUSE, DONATING FABRIC, ELASTIC BANDS, AND OTHER SUPPLIES NECESSARY FOR MASK PRODUCTION. THE INITIATIVE CREATED A SENSE OF CAMARADERIE AND SHARED PURPOSE, BRINGING INDIVIDUALS TOGETHER TO ADDRESS A COMMON CHALLENGE.

THROUGH HER DEDICATION, MARIA NOT ONLY PROVIDED ESSENTIAL PROTECTION TO THOSE ON THE FRONT LINES BUT ALSO INSTILLED A SENSE OF COMFORT AND SECURITY WITHIN THE COMMUNITY. HER EFFORTS ALLEVIATED ANXIETY AND FEAR BY ENSURING THAT INDIVIDUALS HAD ACCESS TO A BASIC YET VITAL TOOL FOR THEIR SAFETY.

MARIA'S SEWING INITIATIVE ALSO EXEMPLIFIED THE POWER OF SMALL ACTIONS CREATING A RIPPLE EFFECT. BY STEPPING UP AND UTILIZING HER SKILLS, SHE INSPIRED OTHERS TO DO THE SAME. MANY INDIVIDUALS, EVEN THOSE WITHOUT SEWING EXPERTISE, JOINED THE INITIATIVE BY DONATING FUNDS, ASSISTING

WITH DISTRIBUTION LOGISTICS, OR SPREADING AWARENESS THROUGH SOCIAL MEDIA.

MARIA'S STORY IS A TESTAMENT TO THE STRENGTH OF COMMUNITY AND THE TRANSFORMATIVE POWER OF INDIVIDUAL ACTIONS. HER SEWING INITIATIVE NOT ONLY PROVIDED PHYSICAL PROTECTION BUT ALSO SYMBOLIZED UNITY, COMPASSION, AND RESILIENCE DURING CHALLENGING TIMES. IT SERVES AS A REMINDER THAT EVEN IN THE FACE OF ADVERSITY, ORDINARY INDIVIDUALS HAVE THE POWER TO MAKE AN EXTRAORDINARY IMPACT THROUGH ACTS OF KINDNESS AND SELFLESSNESS.

KEVIN'S TECH SUPPORT FOR SMALL BUSINESSES:

KEVIN, A TECH-SAVVY PROFESSIONAL, DEMONSTRATED AN EXCEPTIONAL SENSE OF EMPATHY AND COMMUNITY SPIRIT DURING THE COVID-19 PANDEMIC BY PROVIDING MUCH-NEEDED TECH SUPPORT TO SMALL BUSINESSES. UNDERSTANDING THE CHALLENGES FACED BY THESE ENTERPRISES IN ADAPTING TO REMOTE WORK AND ONLINE OPERATIONS, KEVIN SELFLESSLY OFFERED HIS EXPERTISE AND ASSISTANCE.

RECOGNIZING THAT MANY SMALL BUSINESSES LACKED THE TECHNICAL RESOURCES AND

KNOWLEDGE TO NAVIGATE THE DIGITAL LANDSCAPE, KEVIN SAW AN OPPORTUNITY TO MAKE A DIFFERENCE. HE GENEROUSLY VOLUNTEERED HIS TIME AND KNOWLEDGE TO HELP THESE BUSINESSES TRANSITION SMOOTHLY TO REMOTE WORK SETUPS, ONLINE COMMUNICATION PLATFORMS, AND DIGITAL MARKETING STRATEGIES.

KEVIN'S TECH SUPPORT FOR SMALL BUSINESSES ENCOMPASSED A WIDE RANGE OF SERVICES. HE PROVIDED GUIDANCE ON SELECTING AND SETTING UP APPROPRIATE SOFTWARE AND HARDWARE FOR REMOTE WORK, HELPING BUSINESS OWNERS AND EMPLOYEES SEAMLESSLY TRANSITION FROM OFFICE TO HOME SETUPS. HE TROUBLESHOOTED TECHNICAL ISSUES, OFFERED

ADVICE ON CYBERSECURITY MEASURES, AND EDUCATED SMALL BUSINESS OWNERS ON BEST PRACTICES FOR ONLINE OPERATIONS.

BEYOND THE TECHNICAL ASPECTS, KEVIN UNDERSTOOD THE IMPORTANCE OF HUMAN CONNECTION AND COLLABORATION. HE ORGANIZED VIRTUAL WORKSHOPS AND TRAINING SESSIONS TO TEACH SMALL BUSINESS OWNERS AND EMPLOYEES HOW TO EFFECTIVELY UTILIZE DIGITAL TOOLS FOR COMMUNICATION, PROJECT MANAGEMENT, AND CUSTOMER ENGAGEMENT. HE PATIENTLY ANSWERED QUESTIONS, PROVIDED STEP-BY-STEP GUIDANCE, AND EMPOWERED THESE BUSINESSES TO HARNESS THE POWER OF TECHNOLOGY.

KEVIN'S EFFORTS EXTENDED BEYOND HIS DIRECT INTERACTIONS WITH SMALL BUSINESS OWNERS. HE CREATED ONLINE RESOURCES, SUCH AS VIDEO TUTORIALS AND INFORMATIONAL GUIDES, TO ENSURE THAT HIS SUPPORT COULD REACH A WIDER AUDIENCE. THESE RESOURCES ADDRESSED COMMON CHALLENGES FACED BY SMALL BUSINESSES DURING THE PANDEMIC AND PROVIDED PRACTICAL SOLUTIONS AND INSIGHTS.

THROUGH HIS DEDICATION AND EXPERTISE, KEVIN BECAME A TRUSTED ADVISOR AND MENTOR TO MANY SMALL BUSINESS OWNERS. HE ALLEVIATED THEIR ANXIETIES, EMPOWERED THEM WITH THE NECESSARY TECH SKILLS, AND INSTILLED CONFIDENCE IN THEIR ABILITY TO

ADAPT AND THRIVE IN A DIGITAL-CENTRIC WORLD.

KEVIN'S TECH SUPPORT NOT ONLY ENABLED SMALL BUSINESSES TO CONTINUE OPERATING DURING A CHALLENGING TIME BUT ALSO PRESERVED JOBS AND LIVELIHOODS WITHIN THE COMMUNITY. BY HELPING THESE BUSINESSES NAVIGATE THE DIGITAL LANDSCAPE, HE PLAYED A CRUCIAL ROLE IN ENSURING THEIR SUSTAINABILITY AND RESILIENCE.

KEVIN'S STORY EXEMPLIFIES THE PROFOUND IMPACT THAT INDIVIDUALS CAN HAVE WHEN THEY SHARE THEIR KNOWLEDGE AND SKILLS FOR THE BETTERMENT OF THEIR COMMUNITY. HIS SELFLESS DEDICATION TO SUPPORTING

SMALL BUSINESSES SHOWCASED THE STRENGTH OF COMMUNITY COLLABORATION AND THE TRANSFORMATIVE POWER OF TECHNOLOGY IN HELPING ENTERPRISES OVERCOME OBSTACLES AND THRIVE IN THE FACE OF ADVERSITY.

SOPHIA'S MENTORSHIP PROGRAM:

SOPHIA, A SEASONED ENTREPRENEUR, EXEMPLIFIED THE POWER OF MENTORSHIP AND COMMUNITY SUPPORT DURING THE COVID-19 PANDEMIC BY ESTABLISHING A MENTORSHIP PROGRAM FOR ASPIRING ENTREPRENEURS. RECOGNIZING THE UNIQUE CHALLENGES FACED BY INDIVIDUALS STARTING BUSINESSES AMIDST THE UNCERTAINTY OF THE PANDEMIC, SOPHIA

EXTENDED A HELPING HAND TO GUIDE AND INSPIRE THESE BUDDING ENTREPRENEURS.

WITH HER WEALTH OF EXPERIENCE, INDUSTRY KNOWLEDGE, AND A GENUINE DESIRE TO GIVE BACK, SOPHIA CREATED A STRUCTURED MENTORSHIP PROGRAM THAT PROVIDED ASPIRING ENTREPRENEURS WITH VALUABLE GUIDANCE, ADVICE, AND SUPPORT. SHE AIMED TO EMPOWER THESE INDIVIDUALS TO NAVIGATE THE COMPLEXITIES OF STARTING A BUSINESS DURING CHALLENGING TIMES.

SOPHIA CAREFULLY SELECTED A DIVERSE GROUP OF MENTEES, ENSURING REPRESENTATION FROM VARIOUS INDUSTRIES AND BACKGROUNDS. THROUGH REGULAR VIRTUAL MEETINGS, SHE

ESTABLISHED A STRONG BOND WITH EACH MENTEE, FOSTERING AN ENVIRONMENT OF TRUST AND OPEN COMMUNICATION.

DURING THE MENTORSHIP PROGRAM, SOPHIA OFFERED HER EXPERTISE ON A RANGE OF TOPICS, INCLUDING BUSINESS PLANNING, MARKET RESEARCH, BRANDING, MARKETING STRATEGIES, AND FINANCIAL MANAGEMENT. SHE SHARED PRACTICAL INSIGHTS, REAL-WORLD EXPERIENCES, AND ACTIONABLE ADVICE TO HELP HER MENTEES OVERCOME OBSTACLES AND MAKE INFORMED DECISIONS.

SOPHIA'S MENTORSHIP PROGRAM WENT BEYOND IMPARTING BUSINESS KNOWLEDGE. SHE RECOGNIZED THE EMOTIONAL TOLL OF

ENTREPRENEURSHIP AND THE IMPACT IT HAD ON THE MENTAL WELL-BEING OF HER MENTEES. SHE PROVIDED EMOTIONAL SUPPORT, ENCOURAGED SELF-CARE PRACTICES, AND EMPHASIZED THE IMPORTANCE OF RESILIENCE AND PERSEVERANCE.

THE MENTORSHIP PROGRAM ALSO INCLUDED NETWORKING OPPORTUNITIES, WHERE MENTEES HAD THE CHANCE TO CONNECT WITH INDUSTRY PROFESSIONALS, POTENTIAL COLLABORATORS, AND FELLOW ENTREPRENEURS. SOPHIA LEVERAGED HER EXTENSIVE NETWORK TO FACILITATE INTRODUCTIONS, PARTNERSHIPS, AND RESOURCE SHARING, FURTHER ENHANCING THE MENTEES' GROWTH AND OPPORTUNITIES.

THE IMPACT OF SOPHIA'S MENTORSHIP PROGRAM WAS PROFOUND. MENTEES GAINED INVALUABLE INSIGHTS, REFINED THEIR BUSINESS STRATEGIES, AND DEVELOPED A DEEPER UNDERSTANDING OF THEIR TARGET MARKETS. THEY FELT EMPOWERED, SUPPORTED, AND INSPIRED BY SOPHIA'S GUIDANCE, WHICH ALLOWED THEM TO NAVIGATE THE UNCERTAINTIES AND CHALLENGES WITH GREATER CONFIDENCE.

SOPHIA'S DEDICATION TO FOSTERING A SENSE OF COMMUNITY AND EMPOWERING OTHERS EXTENDED BEYOND THE MENTORSHIP PROGRAM. SHE ORGANIZED VIRTUAL WORKSHOPS, PANEL DISCUSSIONS, AND NETWORKING EVENTS FOR MENTEES AND

OTHER ASPIRING ENTREPRENEURS TO CONNECT, SHARE KNOWLEDGE, AND LEARN FROM EACH OTHER'S EXPERIENCES.

THROUGH HER MENTORSHIP PROGRAM, SOPHIA CREATED A RIPPLE EFFECT, EMPOWERING A NEW GENERATION OF ENTREPRENEURS AND FOSTERING A SPIRIT OF COLLABORATION AND RESILIENCE WITHIN THE BUSINESS COMMUNITY. HER SELFLESSNESS, LEADERSHIP, AND COMMITMENT TO SUPPORTING OTHERS SHOWCASED THE TRANSFORMATIVE POWER OF MENTORSHIP AND THE INCREDIBLE IMPACT THAT A SINGLE INDIVIDUAL CAN HAVE ON THE JOURNEYS OF MANY.

SOPHIA'S STORY SERVES AS AN INSPIRATION TO BOTH MENTORS AND MENTEES, DEMONSTRATING THE PROFOUND IMPACT THAT MENTORSHIP CAN HAVE ON PERSONAL AND PROFESSIONAL GROWTH. HER DEDICATION TO UPLIFTING OTHERS AND HER BELIEF IN THE POTENTIAL OF ASPIRING ENTREPRENEURS HAS LEFT AN INDELIBLE MARK ON THE LIVES OF THOSE SHE MENTORED AND THE WIDER ENTREPRENEURIAL COMMUNITY.

SURVIVAL IN CINEMA AND ENTERTAINMENT INDUSTRY

THE COVID-19 PANDEMIC HAS TAKEN A SIGNIFICANT TOLL ON FILMMAKERS, ACTORS, AND ARTISTS, WHOSE LIVELIHOODS DEPEND ON CREATIVE EXPRESSION AND THE ABILITY TO CONNECT WITH AUDIENCES. THE EMOTIONAL STRUGGLES THEY HAVE FACED DURING THIS TIME CANNOT BE UNDERSTATED.

FOR FILMMAKERS, THE PANDEMIC BROUGHT ABOUT THE CLOSURE OF MOVIE THEATERS AND HALTED PRODUCTION ON MANY PROJECTS. THE ANTICIPATION AND EXCITEMENT OF SHARING THEIR STORIES ON THE BIG SCREEN WERE SUDDENLY REPLACED WITH UNCERTAINTY AND DISAPPOINTMENT. THE EMOTIONAL IMPACT OF DELAYED RELEASES, CANCELED PREMIERES, AND THE INABILITY TO CONNECT WITH AUDIENCES

THROUGH THE CINEMATIC EXPERIENCE WEIGHED HEAVILY ON THEIR HEARTS.

ACTORS, TOO, FACED IMMENSE CHALLENGES AS THE PANDEMIC DISRUPTED THE ENTERTAINMENT INDUSTRY. THE SUSPENSION OF FILM AND TELEVISION PRODUCTIONS MEANT LOST OPPORTUNITIES FOR ROLES AND THE UNCERTAINTY OF WHEN THEY COULD RETURN TO WORK. THE EMOTIONAL TOLL OF BEING AWAY FROM THE CRAFT THEY LOVE, THE CAMARADERIE OF SETS, AND THE THRILL OF PERFORMING FOR AN AUDIENCE LEFT MANY FEELING ISOLATED AND ANXIOUS.

ARTISTS ACROSS VARIOUS MEDIUMS, SUCH AS PAINTERS, SCULPTORS, MUSICIANS, AND

DANCERS, ALSO EXPERIENCED THE EMOTIONAL STRAIN OF THE PANDEMIC. CANCELED EXHIBITIONS, ART SHOWS, CONCERTS, AND PERFORMANCES LEFT THEM WITHOUT PLATFORMS TO SHOWCASE THEIR TALENTS AND CONNECT WITH THEIR AUDIENCES. THE FINANCIAL INSTABILITY AND THE FEAR OF LOSING THEIR ARTISTIC IDENTITY TOOK A TOLL ON THEIR MENTAL AND EMOTIONAL WELL-BEING.

THE EMOTIONAL STRUGGLES FACED BY FILMMAKERS, ACTORS, AND ARTISTS EXTENDED BEYOND THEIR PROFESSIONAL LIVES. MANY FOUND THEMSELVES GRAPPLING WITH FINANCIAL INSECURITY, AS GIGS, CONTRACTS, AND FREELANCE OPPORTUNITIES DIMINISHED

OR DISAPPEARED ALTOGETHER. THE PRESSURE TO FIND ALTERNATIVE SOURCES OF INCOME WHILE STAYING TRUE TO THEIR CREATIVE PURSUITS ADDED ANOTHER LAYER OF STRESS AND ANXIETY.

MOREOVER, THE SENSE OF ISOLATION AND DISCONNECTION FROM THEIR ARTISTIC COMMUNITIES WAS DEEPLY FELT. COLLABORATIVE PROJECTS, REHEARSALS, AND CREATIVE BRAINSTORMING SESSIONS, WHICH THRIVE ON PERSONAL INTERACTIONS, WERE ABRUPTLY HALTED. THE ABSENCE OF IN-PERSON CONNECTIONS WITH FELLOW ARTISTS, MENTORS, AND AUDIENCES LEFT A VOID THAT IMPACTED THEIR SENSE OF PURPOSE AND CREATIVE INSPIRATION.

IN THE FACE OF THESE CHALLENGES, HOWEVER, MANY FILMMAKERS, ACTORS, AND ARTISTS HAVE SHOWN IMMENSE RESILIENCE AND DETERMINATION. THEY HAVE FOUND WAYS TO ADAPT, INNOVATE, AND CREATE DESPITE THE CIRCUMSTANCES. VIRTUAL PERFORMANCES, ONLINE EXHIBITIONS, AND COLLABORATIVE PROJECTS CONDUCTED REMOTELY HAVE BECOME A LIFELINE, ALLOWING THEM TO CONTINUE EXPRESSING THEMSELVES AND CONNECTING WITH AUDIENCES IN NEW AND UNCONVENTIONAL WAYS.

FURTHERMORE, THE PANDEMIC HAS SPARKED A RENEWED SENSE OF INTROSPECTION AND EXPLORATION WITHIN THE ARTISTIC COMMUNITY. MANY FILMMAKERS, ACTORS, AND

ARTISTS HAVE USED THIS TIME TO REFLECT ON THEIR CRAFT, EXPERIMENT WITH NEW IDEAS, AND EXPLORE ALTERNATIVE AVENUES OF EXPRESSION. SOME HAVE TAKEN THE OPPORTUNITY TO HONE THEIR SKILLS, ENGAGE IN PERSONAL CREATIVE PROJECTS, AND DELVE DEEPER INTO THEIR ARTISTIC JOURNEYS.

THE EMOTIONAL STRUGGLES FACED BY FILMMAKERS, ACTORS, AND ARTISTS DURING THE PANDEMIC SERVE AS A REMINDER OF THE PROFOUND IMPACT THAT THE ARTS HAVE ON OUR LIVES. THEIR STORIES OF RESILIENCE, ADAPTABILITY, AND UNWAVERING PASSION ARE A TESTAMENT TO THE INDOMITABLE SPIRIT OF THE CREATIVE COMMUNITY. DESPITE THE HARDSHIPS THEY HAVE ENDURED, THEIR

COMMITMENT TO THEIR CRAFT AND THEIR UNWAVERING BELIEF IN THE TRANSFORMATIVE POWER OF ART CONTINUE TO INSPIRE AND UPLIFT US ALL.

THE CINEMA AND ENTERTAINMENT INDUSTRY FACED UNPRECEDENTED CHALLENGES DURING THE COVID-19 PANDEMIC. THE IMPACT OF THE PANDEMIC WAS FELT THROUGHOUT THE ENTIRE ECOSYSTEM OF THE INDUSTRY, AFFECTING FILMMAKERS, ACTORS, PRODUCTION CREWS, DISTRIBUTORS, THEATERS, AND AUDIENCES ALIKE.

1. **FILM PRODUCTION DISRUPTIONS:**

ONE OF THE SIGNIFICANT CHALLENGES

WAS THE SUSPENSION OR DELAY OF FILM PRODUCTIONS WORLDWIDE. TRAVEL RESTRICTIONS, SOCIAL DISTANCING PROTOCOLS, AND SAFETY CONCERNS MADE IT DIFFICULT TO ASSEMBLE CAST AND CREW, FILM ON LOCATION, OR CARRY OUT LARGE-SCALE PRODUCTIONS. MANY PROJECTS HAD TO BE PUT ON HOLD OR MODIFIED TO ADHERE TO HEALTH AND SAFETY GUIDELINES, LEADING TO SCHEDULING CONFLICTS AND FINANCIAL IMPLICATIONS.

2. **CLOSURE OF THEATERS:** MOVIE THEATERS, A VITAL COMPONENT OF THE CINEMA EXPERIENCE, WERE FORCED TO CLOSE THEIR DOORS TO COMPLY WITH

PUBLIC HEALTH MEASURES. THE ABSENCE OF THEATRICAL RELEASES SEVERELY IMPACTED THE REVENUE STREAMS OF PRODUCTION COMPANIES AND DISTRIBUTORS, LEADING TO FINANCIAL LOSSES AND UNCERTAINTY ABOUT THE FUTURE OF THE INDUSTRY.

3. **SHIFT IN CONSUMER BEHAVIOR:** WITH THEATERS CLOSED AND RESTRICTIONS ON PUBLIC GATHERINGS, CONSUMERS TURNED TO ALTERNATIVE FORMS OF ENTERTAINMENT. STREAMING PLATFORMS, VIDEO ON DEMAND, AND AT-HOME MOVIE RELEASES GAINED POPULARITY. THIS SHIFT IN CONSUMER BEHAVIOR ACCELERATED EXISTING

TRENDS TOWARD DIGITAL DISTRIBUTION, CHALLENGING THE TRADITIONAL THEATER MODEL AND RAISING QUESTIONS ABOUT THE FUTURE OF THE CINEMATIC EXPERIENCE.

4. **DISTRIBUTION CHALLENGES:** THE CLOSURE OF THEATERS AND DISRUPTIONS IN FILM FESTIVALS AND INDUSTRY EVENTS CREATED CHALLENGES IN THE DISTRIBUTION OF FILMS. MANY PLANNED RELEASES WERE POSTPONED OR SHIFTED TO DIGITAL PLATFORMS, LEADING TO UNCERTAINTIES REGARDING MARKETING STRATEGIES, AUDIENCE REACH, AND REVENUE GENERATION. INDEPENDENT FILMMAKERS AND SMALLER PRODUCTION

HOUSES FACED PARTICULAR DIFFICULTIES IN SECURING DISTRIBUTION OPPORTUNITIES.

5. **FINANCIAL IMPACT:** THE ECONOMIC DOWNTURN CAUSED BY THE PANDEMIC AFFECTED THE FINANCIAL VIABILITY OF FILM PRODUCTIONS. THE CLOSURE OF THEATERS RESULTED IN REDUCED BOX OFFICE REVENUES, IMPACTING THE PROFITABILITY OF FILMS. THEATRICAL RELEASES OFTEN SERVE AS A CRUCIAL REVENUE DRIVER FOR PRODUCTIONS, AND THE LACK OF THEATRICAL DISTRIBUTION SIGNIFICANTLY IMPACTED THE FINANCIAL STABILITY OF THE INDUSTRY.

6. **UNCERTAINTY AND FEAR:** THE OVERALL UNCERTAINTY SURROUNDING THE PANDEMIC CREATED FEAR AND CAUTION WITHIN THE INDUSTRY. FILMMAKERS, ACTORS, AND INDUSTRY PROFESSIONALS WORRIED ABOUT THEIR HEALTH AND SAFETY ON SET, POTENTIAL DISRUPTIONS TO ONGOING PRODUCTIONS, AND THE VIABILITY OF FUTURE PROJECTS. THE LACK OF CLARITY REGARDING THE TIMELINE FOR THE RETURN OF NORMALCY ADDED TO THE SENSE OF UNEASE AND MADE IT CHALLENGING TO PLAN FOR THE FUTURE.

DESPITE THESE CHALLENGES, THE CINEMA AND ENTERTAINMENT INDUSTRY DEMONSTRATED

RESILIENCE AND ADAPTABILITY. FILMMAKERS EXPLORED ALTERNATIVE PRODUCTION METHODS, SUCH AS REMOTE FILMING AND VIRTUAL COLLABORATIONS. STREAMING PLATFORMS AND DIGITAL RELEASES PROVIDED NEW AVENUES FOR FILMMAKERS TO REACH AUDIENCES DIRECTLY. DRIVE-IN THEATERS EXPERIENCED A RESURGENCE, OFFERING A SOCIALLY DISTANCED CINEMATIC EXPERIENCE. INDUSTRY PROFESSIONALS WORKED TOGETHER TO DEVELOP HEALTH AND SAFETY PROTOCOLS TO ENABLE THE RESUMPTION OF PRODUCTION ACTIVITIES.

THE CHALLENGES FACED BY THE CINEMA AND ENTERTAINMENT INDUSTRY DURING THE PANDEMIC HAVE HIGHLIGHTED THE NEED FOR

INNOVATION, FLEXIBILITY, AND COLLABORATION. THE INDUSTRY CONTINUES TO EVOLVE, EMBRACING NEW DISTRIBUTION MODELS, DIGITAL TECHNOLOGIES, AND CREATIVE APPROACHES TO STORYTELLING. AS THE WORLD RECOVERS FROM THE PANDEMIC, THE CINEMA AND ENTERTAINMENT INDUSTRY WILL CONTINUE TO ADAPT AND FIND WAYS TO ENTERTAIN, INSPIRE, AND CONNECT WITH AUDIENCES.

EMILY'S VIRTUAL THEATER PRODUCTION:

EMILY, A THEATER DIRECTOR, REFUSED TO LET THE LIMITATIONS OF THE PANDEMIC DAMPEN HER CREATIVITY AND LOVE FOR THE STAGE. DETERMINED TO BRING THE MAGIC OF

THEATER TO AUDIENCES DESPITE THE RESTRICTIONS ON LIVE PERFORMANCES, SHE EMBARKED ON A JOURNEY TO CREATE A VIRTUAL THEATER PRODUCTION.

GATHERING A TALENTED ENSEMBLE OF ACTORS, EMILY COORDINATED REHEARSALS AND SCRIPT READINGS VIA VIDEO CONFERENCING PLATFORMS. DESPITE BEING PHYSICALLY SCATTERED ACROSS DIFFERENT LOCATIONS, THE CAST EMBRACED THE CHALLENGE, IMMERSING THEMSELVES IN THEIR CHARACTERS AND DELIVERING POWERFUL PERFORMANCES THROUGH THEIR SCREENS.

UTILIZING VIDEO EDITING TECHNIQUES, GREEN SCREENS, AND CREATIVE SET DESIGNS, EMILY TRANSFORMED EACH ACTOR'S INDIVIDUAL RECORDINGS INTO A SEAMLESS PRODUCTION. WITH CAREFUL ATTENTION TO DETAIL, SHE SYNCHRONIZED THEIR PERFORMANCES, INTEGRATING VISUAL EFFECTS AND SOUNDSCAPES TO REPLICATE THE AMBIANCE OF A LIVE THEATER EXPERIENCE.

WHEN THE VIRTUAL PRODUCTION PREMIERED, AUDIENCES WERE CAPTIVATED BY THE INGENUITY AND PASSION THAT WENT INTO ITS CREATION. THE POWER OF THE PERFORMANCES TRANSCENDED THE PHYSICAL DISTANCE, TOUCHING THE HEARTS OF VIEWERS WHO FOUND SOLACE AND INSPIRATION IN THE ARTISTRY AND RESILIENCE OF THE CAST AND CREW.

MIGUEL'S ONLINE ART EXHIBITION

MIGUEL, A VISUAL ARTIST, HAD LONG DREAMED OF HOLDING A SOLO EXHIBITION TO SHOWCASE HIS UNIQUE CREATIONS. WHEN TRADITIONAL GALLERY SPACES BECAME INACCESSIBLE DUE TO THE PANDEMIC, HE TURNED TO THE DIGITAL REALM TO BRING HIS ARTWORK TO LIFE.

WITH METICULOUS PLANNING AND THE SUPPORT OF A DEDICATED TEAM, MIGUEL CURATED AN ONLINE ART EXHIBITION THAT REPLICATED THE IMMERSIVE EXPERIENCE OF VISITING A PHYSICAL GALLERY. THROUGH A

VIRTUAL TOUR, VIEWERS COULD NAVIGATE THROUGH DIFFERENT ROOMS, ZOOM IN ON INDIVIDUAL PIECES, AND READ DESCRIPTIONS ABOUT EACH ARTWORK.

TO ENHANCE THE INTERACTIVE EXPERIENCE, MIGUEL INCORPORATED MULTIMEDIA ELEMENTS. VIEWERS COULD LISTEN TO AUDIO RECORDINGS OF THE ARTIST DISCUSSING HIS CREATIVE PROCESS, WATCH BEHIND-THE-SCENES VIDEOS, AND EVEN ENGAGE IN LIVE CHATS WITH MIGUEL HIMSELF DURING SCHEDULED ONLINE EVENTS.

THE ONLINE EXHIBITION ALLOWED MIGUEL TO REACH A WIDER AUDIENCE BEYOND THE CONSTRAINTS OF A PHYSICAL LOCATION. ART ENTHUSIASTS FROM DIFFERENT PARTS OF THE WORLD COULD EXPLORE AND APPRECIATE HIS WORK, FOSTERING CONNECTIONS AND CONVERSATIONS THAT TRANSCENDED BORDERS AND TIME ZONES.

SOFIA'S MUSIC COLLABORATION:

SOFIA, A MUSICIAN AND SONGWRITER, FOUND SOLACE IN THE POWER OF VIRTUAL COLLABORATIONS DURING THE ISOLATING TIMES OF THE PANDEMIC. DETERMINED TO CREATE MUSIC AND CONNECT WITH FELLOW MUSICIANS DESPITE THE PHYSICAL DISTANCE, SHE INITIATED A COLLABORATIVE PROJECT THAT SPANNED MULTIPLE COUNTRIES.

USING VIDEO CONFERENCING SOFTWARE, SOFIA GATHERED MUSICIANS FROM DIFFERENT BACKGROUNDS AND CULTURES, EACH CONTRIBUTING THEIR UNIQUE MUSICAL TALENTS TO THE PROJECT. FROM INSTRUMENTALISTS TO VOCALISTS, THEY SHARED THEIR RECORDINGS AND IDEAS, SEAMLESSLY WEAVING THEIR INDIVIDUAL PERFORMANCES INTO A HARMONIOUS AND COHESIVE COMPOSITION.

AS THE MUSIC TOOK SHAPE, SOFIA AND HER COLLABORATORS ALSO EXPLORED INNOVATIVE WAYS TO VISUALLY REPRESENT THEIR COLLABORATION. THEY EXCHANGED VIDEO CLIPS OF THEMSELVES PERFORMING, WHICH

WERE EDITED TOGETHER TO CREATE A VISUALLY CAPTIVATING MUSIC VIDEO THAT SHOWCASED THEIR COLLECTIVE TALENT AND DEDICATION.

THE FINAL RESULT WAS A STUNNING MUSICAL CREATION THAT REFLECTED THE UNITY AND RESILIENCE OF THE ARTISTS INVOLVED. THE COLLABORATIVE PROJECT NOT ONLY BROUGHT JOY AND INSPIRATION TO THE MUSICIANS THEMSELVES BUT ALSO TOUCHED THE HEARTS OF LISTENERS AROUND THE WORLD, REMINDING THEM OF THE POWER OF MUSIC TO UPLIFT AND HEAL.

EMMA'S FILM:

IN THE FACE OF THE COVID-19 PANDEMIC, A YOUNG ASPIRING FILMMAKER NAMED EMMA FOUND HERSELF NAVIGATING UNCHARTED TERRITORY. WITH FILM SCHOOLS CLOSED,

PRODUCTION HALTED, AND INDUSTRY EVENTS CANCELED, HER DREAMS OF MAKING HER FIRST SHORT FILM SEEMED TO BE SLIPPING AWAY. HOWEVER, EMMA REFUSED TO LET THE CIRCUMSTANCES CRUSH HER SPIRIT. INSTEAD, SHE EMBRACED THE CHALLENGES AND EMBARKED ON A JOURNEY OF CREATIVE RESILIENCE.

UNDETERRED BY THE LIMITATIONS, EMMA DECIDED TO HARNESS THE POWER OF VIRTUAL COLLABORATIONS. SHE REACHED OUT TO FELLOW FILMMAKERS, ACTORS, AND ARTISTS, INVITING THEM TO JOIN HER IN BRINGING HER SCRIPT TO LIFE. THROUGH VIDEO CONFERENCING, THEY DISCUSSED IDEAS,

DEVELOPED THE CHARACTERS, AND DESIGNED THE VISUAL AESTHETICS OF THE FILM.

WITH A COMMITTED CAST AND CREW ASSEMBLED, THE NEXT OBSTACLE WAS FIGURING OUT HOW TO SHOOT THE FILM WHILE ADHERING TO THE SAFETY PROTOCOLS. EMMA CAME UP WITH AN INGENIOUS PLAN: A REMOTE SHOOTING PROCESS. EACH ACTOR WOULD FILM THEIR SCENES INDIVIDUALLY USING THEIR SMARTPHONES OR CAMERAS, FOLLOWING THE GUIDELINES AND DIRECTIONS PROVIDED BY EMMA.

THIS VIRTUAL PRODUCTION REQUIRED METICULOUS PLANNING AND COORDINATION. EMMA CONDUCTED VIRTUAL REHEARSALS,

GUIDING THE ACTORS THROUGH THEIR PERFORMANCES, AND OFFERING FEEDBACK TO ENSURE THE DESIRED EMOTIONAL IMPACT. THE ACTORS TRANSFORMED THEIR HOMES INTO SETS, IMPROVISING PROPS AND COSTUMES TO BRING AUTHENTICITY TO THEIR CHARACTERS.

WHILE THE PHYSICAL DISTANCE PRESENTED CHALLENGES, EMMA DISCOVERED THAT IT ALSO OPENED UP OPPORTUNITIES FOR CREATIVITY. SHE EXPERIMENTED WITH DIFFERENT ANGLES, LIGHTING TECHNIQUES, AND EDITING STYLES TO CREATE A VISUALLY COMPELLING NARRATIVE. THROUGH INNOVATIVE EDITING AND POST-PRODUCTION TECHNIQUES, SHE SEAMLESSLY WEAVED TOGETHER THE ACTORS'

INDIVIDUAL FOOTAGE, CRAFTING A COHESIVE STORY.

EMMA'S DETERMINATION AND RESOURCEFULNESS PAID OFF AS HER FILM STARTED TO TAKE SHAPE. SHE ENLISTED THE HELP OF A TALENTED COMPOSER WHO CREATED AN EVOCATIVE MUSICAL SCORE TO ENHANCE THE EMOTIONAL DEPTH OF THE STORY. SOUND DESIGNERS AND VISUAL EFFECTS ARTISTS ADDED THEIR MAGIC, BRINGING A CINEMATIC QUALITY TO THE FINAL PRODUCT.

WHEN THE FILM WAS COMPLETED, EMMA ORGANIZED A VIRTUAL PREMIERE FOR HER CAST, CREW, AND FRIENDS. DESPITE NOT BEING PHYSICALLY TOGETHER, THE SENSE OF

ANTICIPATION AND EXCITEMENT FILLED THE VIRTUAL SPACE. AS THE FILM PLAYED, EMMA'S HEART SWELLED WITH PRIDE. THE STORY SHE HAD ENVISIONED HAD COME TO LIFE, TRANSCENDING THE LIMITATIONS OF THE PANDEMIC.

THE FILM RESONATED DEEPLY WITH THE AUDIENCE, NOT ONLY FOR ITS COMPELLING STORY BUT ALSO FOR THE COLLECTIVE EFFORT AND RESILIENCE IT REPRESENTED. EMMA'S JOURNEY INSPIRED OTHER ASPIRING FILMMAKERS TO EMBRACE CREATIVITY IN THE FACE OF ADVERSITY AND TO FIND INNOVATIVE WAYS TO PURSUE THEIR DREAMS.

AS EMMA'S FILM GAINED RECOGNITION THROUGH ONLINE FILM FESTIVALS AND DIGITAL PLATFORMS, IT BECAME A TESTAMENT TO THE POWER OF ART TO UPLIFT AND HEAL. AUDIENCES FOUND SOLACE, ESCAPISM, AND CONNECTION THROUGH HER STORYTELLING, REMINDING THEM OF THE RESILIENCE OF THE HUMAN SPIRIT AND THE CAPACITY OF ART TO TRANSCEND BARRIERS.

EMMA'S JOURNEY FROM SCRIPT TO SCREEN PROVED THAT PASSION, CREATIVITY, AND COLLABORATION CAN OVERCOME EVEN THE MOST CHALLENGING CIRCUMSTANCES. HER STORY SERVES AS A BEACON OF HOPE FOR ASPIRING FILMMAKERS WORLDWIDE, REMINDING THEM THAT WITH

DETERMINATION, INGENUITY, AND A BELIEF IN THEIR VISION, DREAMS CAN BECOME A REALITY, NO MATTER THE OBSTACLES IN THEIR PATH.

THESE STORIES EXEMPLIFY THE CREATIVE RESILIENCE, VIRTUAL COLLABORATIONS, AND THE TRANSFORMATIVE POWER OF ART DURING CHALLENGING TIMES. DESPITE THE LIMITATIONS IMPOSED BY THE PANDEMIC, ARTISTS LIKE EMILY, MIGUEL, AND SOFIA FOUND INNOVATIVE WAYS TO SHARE THEIR PASSION, CONNECT WITH OTHERS, AND BRING JOY AND INSPIRATION TO AUDIENCES. THEIR STORIES SERVE AS A TESTAMENT TO THE ENDURING SPIRIT OF CREATIVITY AND THE ABILITY OF ART TO UPLIFT, HEAL, AND UNITE US, EVEN IN THE FACE OF ADVERSITY.

SPORTS AND ATHLETES

THE WORLD OF SPORTS WAS ABRUPTLY HALTED BY THE COVID-19 PANDEMIC, LEAVING ATHLETES STRANDED IN A WHIRLWIND OF EMOTIONS AS COMPETITIONS WERE CANCELED, DREAMS WERE SHATTERED, AND THEIR RELENTLESS PURSUIT OF GREATNESS WAS PUT ON HOLD. THE ROLLERCOASTER OF EMOTIONS EXPERIENCED BY THESE ATHLETES WAS LIKE NO OTHER, AS THEY GRAPPLED WITH DISAPPOINTMENT, FRUSTRATION, AND A PROFOUND SENSE OF LOSS.

1. **ANTICIPATION AND PREPARATION:** ATHLETES HAD BEEN

DILIGENTLY PREPARING FOR UPCOMING COMPETITIONS, INVESTING COUNTLESS HOURS IN TRAINING, PUSHING THEIR BODIES TO THE LIMITS, AND FINE-TUNING THEIR SKILLS. THE EXCITEMENT AND ANTICIPATION WERE PALPABLE AS THEY ENVISIONED STEPPING ONTO THE FIELD, COURT, OR TRACK TO SHOWCASE THEIR TALENT AND COMPETE AGAINST THE BEST. THE COMMITMENT AND SACRIFICES MADE TO REACH PEAK PERFORMANCE WERE ALL-CONSUMING.

2. **SHOCK AND DISBELIEF:** WHEN NEWS OF COMPETITION CANCELLATIONS AND POSTPONEMENTS HIT, ATHLETES WERE LEFT STUNNED AND IN DISBELIEF. THEIR DREAMS WERE SUDDENLY SHATTERED, AND THE CULMINATION OF THEIR HARD WORK SEEMED TO SLIP AWAY. THE INITIAL SHOCK GAVE WAY TO A FLOOD OF EMOTIONS AS THEY TRIED TO PROCESS THE SUDDEN CHANGE IN THEIR ATHLETIC

JOURNEY.

3. **GRIEF AND LOSS:** THE CANCELED COMPETITIONS REPRESENTED MORE THAN JUST MISSED OPPORTUNITIES. ATHLETES MOURNED THE LOSS OF A SEASON THEY HAD EAGERLY ANTICIPATED. FOR SOME, IT MEANT THE LOSS OF A CHANCE TO PROVE THEMSELVES, SECURE SCHOLARSHIPS, OR QUALIFY FOR PRESTIGIOUS EVENTS. THE WEIGHT OF DISAPPOINTMENT SETTLED HEAVILY ON THEIR SHOULDERS, LEAVING THEM TO GRAPPLE WITH THE VOID LEFT BY UNFULFILLED DREAMS.

4. **FRUSTRATION AND ANGER:** ATHLETES FACED IMMENSE FRUSTRATION AND ANGER AS THEY NAVIGATED THE UNCERTAINTY AND LACK OF CONTROL BROUGHT ON BY THE PANDEMIC. THE SUDDEN DISRUPTION TO THEIR TRAINING ROUTINES, THE INABILITY TO COMPETE, AND THE LOSS OF CAMARADERIE WITH

TEAMMATES ADDED FUEL TO THEIR EMOTIONAL ROLLERCOASTER. THE ANGER AT CIRCUMSTANCES BEYOND THEIR CONTROL FUELED A DETERMINATION TO RISE ABOVE THE CHALLENGES AND FIND ALTERNATIVE WAYS TO STAY CONNECTED TO THEIR SPORT.

5. **RESILIENCE AND ADAPTATION:** AMIDST THE TURMOIL, ATHLETES DEMONSTRATED REMARKABLE RESILIENCE. THEY QUICKLY ADAPTED THEIR TRAINING ROUTINES, FINDING WAYS TO STAY FIT AND MAINTAIN THEIR FOCUS DESPITE LIMITED RESOURCES AND TRAINING FACILITIES. THEY EXPLORED VIRTUAL TRAINING SESSIONS, ENGAGED IN HOME WORKOUTS, AND SOUGHT CREATIVE WAYS TO SIMULATE COMPETITION EXPERIENCES. THIS RESILIENCE BECAME A TESTAMENT TO THEIR UNWAVERING DEDICATION AND

THEIR ABILITY TO PIVOT IN THE FACE OF ADVERSITY.

6. **HOPE AND RENEWED PURPOSE:** AS TIME WENT ON, ATHLETES FOUND GLIMMERS OF HOPE. THEY BEGAN TO REDEFINE THEIR GOALS, SHIFTING THEIR FOCUS FROM IMMEDIATE COMPETITIONS TO LONG-TERM DEVELOPMENT. THE FORCED BREAK ALLOWED THEM TO REFLECT, REASSESS THEIR STRENGTHS AND WEAKNESSES, AND WORK ON ASPECTS OF THEIR PERFORMANCE THAT WERE OFTEN OVERLOOKED. THEY DISCOVERED RENEWED PURPOSE, FINDING SOLACE IN THE FACT THAT THEIR DEDICATION TO THEIR SPORT WOULD ENDURE, NO MATTER THE CIRCUMSTANCES.

7. **VIRTUAL CONNECTIONS AND SUPPORT:** ATHLETES LEANED ON EACH OTHER FOR SUPPORT, FORGING VIRTUAL CONNECTIONS WITH TEAMMATES, COACHES, AND FELLOW ATHLETES. THEY FOUND SOLACE IN SHARING THEIR STRUGGLES, EXCHANGING TRAINING TIPS, AND OFFERING WORDS OF ENCOURAGEMENT. ONLINE PLATFORMS BECAME A LIFELINE, ALLOWING ATHLETES TO STAY CONNECTED TO THEIR SPORTING COMMUNITIES AND MAINTAIN A SENSE OF CAMARADERIE DESPITE PHYSICAL DISTANCE.

8. **RETURN TO COMPETITION:** AS RESTRICTIONS EASED AND COMPETITIONS SLOWLY RESUMED, ATHLETES EXPERIENCED A MIX OF EXCITEMENT AND APPREHENSION. THE RETURN TO THE FIELD BROUGHT A SURGE OF EMOTIONS—NERVOUSNESS,

ANTICIPATION, AND A RENEWED SENSE OF PURPOSE. STEPPING BACK INTO THE ARENA, THEY WERE REMINDED OF THEIR LOVE FOR THE SPORT AND THEIR UNYIELDING DESIRE TO EXCEL.

THE EMOTIONAL ROLLERCOASTER EXPERIENCED BY ATHLETES DURING THE PANDEMIC WAS A TESTAMENT TO THEIR PASSION, RESILIENCE, AND UNWAVERING DEDICATION. THROUGH THE HIGHS AND LOWS, THEY LEARNED THE VALUE OF ADAPTABILITY, PERSEVERANCE, AND THE IMPORTANCE OF FINDING STRENGTH IN THE FACE OF ADVERSITY.

EMILY'S OLYMPIC DREAM:

EMILY, A YOUNG GYMNAST, HAD BEEN TRAINING TIRELESSLY FOR YEARS WITH ONE GOAL IN MIND—TO REPRESENT HER COUNTRY IN THE OLYMPIC GAMES. HOWEVER, WHEN THE PANDEMIC HIT AND THE GAMES WERE POSTPONED, EMILY'S DREAMS WERE SUDDENLY PUT ON HOLD. INSTEAD OF GIVING UP, SHE DOUBLED DOWN ON HER TRAINING, MAINTAINING HER DISCIPLINE AND UNWAVERING FOCUS.

WITH GYMS CLOSED, EMILY CONVERTED HER GARAGE INTO A TRAINING SPACE. SHE IMPROVISED WITH HOUSEHOLD ITEMS, USING CHAIRS AS MAKESHIFT BALANCE BEAMS AND CUSHIONS AS LANDING MATS. SHE SET UP A VIDEO CALL WITH HER COACH, WHO GUIDED HER THROUGH VIRTUAL TRAINING SESSIONS, ENSURING THAT SHE CONTINUED TO REFINE HER ROUTINES AND TECHNIQUES.

EMILY FACED NUMEROUS SETBACKS, BATTLING INJURIES AND MOMENTS OF DOUBT ALONG THE

WAY. BUT HER DETERMINATION WAS UNYIELDING. SHE REFUSED TO LET THE CIRCUMSTANCES DETER HER FROM HER OLYMPIC DREAM. SHE SOUGHT INSPIRATION FROM PAST GYMNASTICS CHAMPIONS, WATCHING THEIR PERFORMANCES AND STUDYING THEIR TECHNIQUES TO FURTHER IMPROVE HER SKILLS.

WHEN THE OLYMPIC GAMES FINALLY ARRIVED A YEAR LATER, EMILY STOOD ON THE WORLD STAGE, READY TO SHOWCASE HER TALENT AND RESILIENCE. DESPITE THE CHALLENGES SHE HAD FACED, SHE EXECUTED HER ROUTINES FLAWLESSLY, CAPTIVATING THE AUDIENCE WITH HER GRACE AND STRENGTH. WHILE SHE DIDN'T WIN A MEDAL, HER STORY INSPIRED MILLIONS, REMINDING THEM OF THE POWER OF PERSEVERANCE AND THE INDOMITABLE HUMAN SPIRIT IN SPORTS.

CARLOS'S COMEBACK:

CARLOS, A PROFESSIONAL SOCCER PLAYER, FACED A DEVASTATING SETBACK WHEN HE SUFFERED A CAREER-THREATENING INJURY DURING A CRUCIAL MATCH JUST BEFORE THE PANDEMIC STRUCK. THE MONTHS OF REHABILITATION AND UNCERTAINTY THAT FOLLOWED TESTED HIS MENTAL AND PHYSICAL STRENGTH. BUT CARLOS REFUSED TO LET HIS INJURY DEFINE HIM.

WITH THE HELP OF A DEDICATED TEAM OF DOCTORS, PHYSIOTHERAPISTS, AND TRAINERS, CARLOS EMBARKED ON A GRUELING RECOVERY JOURNEY. EVERY DAY WAS A BATTLE AGAINST PAIN AND DOUBT, BUT HE REMAINED FOCUSED ON HIS ULTIMATE GOAL—TO RETURN TO THE FIELD AND PLAY THE SPORT HE LOVED.

DURING THE PANDEMIC, CARLOS FOUND SOLACE IN THE SOLITUDE OF HIS TRAINING SESSIONS. HE PUSHED HIS BODY TO ITS LIMITS, GRADUALLY REGAINING HIS STRENGTH AND AGILITY. VIRTUAL SESSIONS WITH HIS TEAMMATES AND COACHES KEPT HIM

CONNECTED TO THE SPORT AND PROVIDED INVALUABLE SUPPORT AND MOTIVATION.

AS RESTRICTIONS EASED AND COMPETITIONS RESUMED, CARLOS MADE HIS LONG-AWAITED COMEBACK. THE MOMENT HE STEPPED ONTO THE FIELD, A SURGE OF EMOTIONS OVERWHELMED HIM. THE CHEERS OF THE CROWD FILLED HIS EARS, FUELING HIS DETERMINATION TO PROVE THAT HE WAS STRONGER THAN EVER.

CARLOS'S RETURN WAS NOTHING SHORT OF REMARKABLE. HE DISPLAYED A LEVEL OF SKILL AND RESILIENCE THAT ASTONISHED BOTH TEAMMATES AND OPPONENTS. WITH EACH GAME, HE REMINDED THE WORLD THAT SETBACKS ARE JUST TEMPORARY OBSTACLES, AND TRUE CHAMPIONS RISE ABOVE THEM.

HIS COMEBACK STORY BECAME AN INSPIRATION FOR ATHLETES AND FANS ALIKE, DEMONSTRATING THE POWER OF THE HUMAN SPIRIT TO OVERCOME ADVERSITY AND ACHIEVE GREATNESS. CARLOS'S JOURNEY TAUGHT

EVERYONE THAT WITH UNWAVERING DETERMINATION, RELENTLESS HARD WORK, AND A REFUSAL TO GIVE UP, DREAMS CAN BE REALIZED EVEN IN THE FACE OF THE MOST CHALLENGING CIRCUMSTANCES.

ANNA'S MARATHON TRIUMPH:

ANNA, AN AMATEUR RUNNER, HAD BEEN TRAINING FOR HER FIRST MARATHON WHEN THE PANDEMIC DISRUPTED THE ENTIRE RACING CALENDAR. HER MONTHS OF PREPARATION AND DEDICATION WERE SUDDENLY UPENDED, LEAVING HER FEELING DISHEARTENED AND UNCERTAIN ABOUT THE FUTURE.

RATHER THAN SUCCUMBING TO DESPAIR, ANNA DECIDED TO CHANNEL HER ENERGY INTO SOMETHING POSITIVE. SHE CONTINUED HER TRAINING REGIMEN, EXPLORING NEW ROUTES IN HER NEIGHBORHOOD AND EMBRACING VIRTUAL RACES. SHE CONNECTED WITH A GLOBAL COMMUNITY OF RUNNERS WHO SHARED HER PASSION, PARTICIPATING IN

VIRTUAL MARATHONS THAT ALLOWED HER TO COMPETE FROM A DISTANCE.

ANNA'S DETERMINATION TO CONQUER THE MARATHON DISTANCE REMAINED UNWAVERING. WHEN IN-PERSON RACES RESUMED, SHE SEIZED THE OPPORTUNITY. WITH STRICT SAFETY PROTOCOLS IN PLACE, ANNA JOINED FELLOW RUNNERS AT THE STARTING LINE, FUELED BY THE MONTHS

GENDER PERSPECTIVES: MEN AND WOMEN

DURING THE COVID-19 PANDEMIC, BOTH MEN AND WOMEN EXPERIENCED A RANGE OF EMOTIONAL IMPACTS AS THEY GRAPPLED WITH THE BURDENS OF CAREGIVING, DOMESTIC VIOLENCE, AND MENTAL HEALTH CHALLENGES. THE PANDEMIC AMPLIFIED PRE-EXISTING SOCIETAL ISSUES AND PLACED ADDITIONAL STRAIN ON INDIVIDUALS AND FAMILIES, AFFECTING THEIR EMOTIONAL WELL-BEING IN PROFOUND WAYS.

1. **CAREGIVING RESPONSIBILITIES:** WITH SCHOOLS AND DAYCARE CENTERS CLOSED, MANY FAMILIES FOUND THEMSELVES NAVIGATING THE CHALLENGES OF WORKING FROM HOME WHILE TAKING CARE OF CHILDREN AND ELDERLY FAMILY MEMBERS. BOTH MEN AND WOMEN FACED INCREASED RESPONSIBILITIES IN MANAGING HOUSEHOLD CHORES, HOMESCHOOLING, AND PROVIDING EMOTIONAL SUPPORT. THE EMOTIONAL TOLL OF JUGGLING MULTIPLE ROLES AND THE PRESSURE TO MEET EVERYONE'S NEEDS WEIGHED HEAVILY ON CAREGIVERS, LEADING TO STRESS, EXHAUSTION, AND FEELINGS OF BEING OVERWHELMED.

2. **DOMESTIC VIOLENCE:** THE PANDEMIC HEIGHTENED THE RISK OF DOMESTIC VIOLENCE, WITH VICTIMS FACING PROLONGED PERIODS OF ISOLATION AND LIMITED ACCESS TO

SUPPORT NETWORKS. BOTH MEN AND WOMEN EXPERIENCED THE EMOTIONAL TURMOIL OF LIVING IN FEAR AND UNCERTAINTY WITHIN THEIR OWN HOMES. SURVIVORS STRUGGLED WITH THE DIFFICULT DECISION OF SEEKING HELP AND BREAKING FREE FROM ABUSIVE SITUATIONS, OFTEN COMPOUNDED BY FINANCIAL CONSTRAINTS AND THE LACK OF SAFE SPACES DURING LOCKDOWNS.

3. **MENTAL HEALTH CHALLENGES:** THE PANDEMIC BROUGHT A SURGE IN MENTAL HEALTH ISSUES FOR BOTH MEN AND WOMEN. THE STRESS, FEAR, AND SOCIAL ISOLATION TRIGGERED FEELINGS OF ANXIETY, DEPRESSION, AND LONELINESS. MEN, IN PARTICULAR, FACED SOCIETAL PRESSURES THAT DISCOURAGED THEM FROM SEEKING HELP AND EXPRESSING VULNERABILITY. WOMEN, ON THE OTHER HAND, CARRIED THE EMOTIONAL WEIGHT OF CARETAKING,

OFTEN PUTTING THEIR OWN MENTAL HEALTH NEEDS ON THE BACKBURNER. ACCESS TO MENTAL HEALTH SUPPORT AND RESOURCES BECAME CRUCIAL IN ADDRESSING THESE CHALLENGES.

4. **EMOTIONAL EXHAUSTION:** MEN AND WOMEN ALIKE EXPERIENCED EMOTIONAL EXHAUSTION AS THEY NAVIGATED THE UNCERTAINTIES AND CONSTANT CHANGES BROUGHT ON BY THE PANDEMIC. THE CONSTANT BARRAGE OF DISTRESSING NEWS, FINANCIAL WORRIES, AND CONCERNS FOR THE HEALTH AND SAFETY OF LOVED ONES TOOK A TOLL ON THEIR EMOTIONAL WELL-BEING. MANY STRUGGLED TO FIND MOMENTS OF RESPITE AND SELF-CARE IN AN ENVIRONMENT THAT FELT RELENTLESSLY DEMANDING.

5. **RESILIENCE AND SUPPORT:** DESPITE THE CHALLENGES, INDIVIDUALS DEMONSTRATED REMARKABLE RESILIENCE IN THE FACE OF ADVERSITY. MEN AND WOMEN SOUGHT SUPPORT FROM THEIR SOCIAL NETWORKS, ENGAGING IN VIRTUAL GATHERINGS, AND SHARING THEIR EXPERIENCES TO FOSTER CONNECTION AND EMPATHY. COMMUNITIES RALLIED TOGETHER TO PROVIDE RESOURCES AND EMOTIONAL SUPPORT, RECOGNIZING THE IMPORTANCE OF COLLECTIVE RESILIENCE.

6. **ADVOCACY AND AWARENESS:** THE PANDEMIC ALSO SPURRED CONVERSATIONS AROUND GENDER ROLES, DOMESTIC VIOLENCE, AND MENTAL HEALTH, PROMPTING A GREATER RECOGNITION OF THE NEED FOR SYSTEMIC CHANGE. MEN AND WOMEN JOINED FORCES TO ADVOCATE FOR BETTER SUPPORT SYSTEMS, INCREASED

ACCESS TO MENTAL HEALTH SERVICES, AND RESOURCES TO ADDRESS DOMESTIC VIOLENCE. THIS COLLECTIVE EFFORT HELPED TO RAISE AWARENESS AND BREAK THE SILENCE SURROUNDING THESE CRITICAL ISSUES.

IT IS CRUCIAL TO ACKNOWLEDGE AND ADDRESS THE EMOTIONAL IMPACT OF CAREGIVING RESPONSIBILITIES, DOMESTIC VIOLENCE, AND MENTAL HEALTH CHALLENGES ON BOTH MEN AND WOMEN DURING THE PANDEMIC. BY FOSTERING OPEN DIALOGUE, PROMOTING SUPPORT NETWORKS, AND ADVOCATING FOR COMPREHENSIVE POLICIES, SOCIETIES CAN WORK TOWARDS CREATING A MORE INCLUSIVE

AND EMPATHETIC ENVIRONMENT THAT PRIORITIZES EMOTIONAL WELL-BEING FOR ALL.

EMMA'S COMMUNITY KITCHEN:

WHEN THE PANDEMIC HIT, EMMA, A RESTAURANT OWNER, WAS FACED WITH THE DEVASTATING REALITY OF HAVING TO CLOSE HER BUSINESS. INSTEAD OF SUCCUMBING TO DESPAIR, SHE CHANNELED HER ENERGY INTO HELPING OTHERS. EMMA TRANSFORMED HER RESTAURANT INTO A COMMUNITY KITCHEN, PROVIDING FREE MEALS TO THOSE IN NEED.

WORD QUICKLY SPREAD ABOUT EMMA'S INITIATIVE, AND SOON VOLUNTEERS STARTED JOINING HER CAUSE. PEOPLE FROM ALL WALKS OF LIFE CAME TOGETHER, OFFERING THEIR TIME AND RESOURCES TO ENSURE THAT NOBODY IN THEIR COMMUNITY WENT HUNGRY. THE KITCHEN BECAME A HUB OF COMPASSION AND SUPPORT, WHERE INDIVIDUALS NOT ONLY RECEIVED NOURISHMENT BUT ALSO FOUND SOLACE AND CONNECTION DURING CHALLENGING TIMES.

EMMA'S ACT OF KINDNESS AND HER ABILITY TO RALLY HER COMMUNITY INSPIRED OTHERS TO DO THE SAME. SOON, SIMILAR INITIATIVES POPPED UP IN NEIGHBORING TOWNS, CREATING A NETWORK OF COMMUNITY KITCHENS THAT

PROVIDED FOOD, COMFORT, AND A SENSE OF BELONGING TO THOSE IN NEED. THROUGH HER STRENGTH AND COMPASSION, EMMA SHOWED THAT EVEN IN THE DARKEST TIMES, THE HUMAN SPIRIT CAN SHINE THROUGH AND MAKE A POSITIVE IMPACT ON THE LIVES OF OTHERS.

MARK'S SUPPORT GROUP:

MARK, A MENTAL HEALTH ADVOCATE, RECOGNIZED THE INCREASED NEED FOR EMOTIONAL SUPPORT DURING THE PANDEMIC. HE STARTED A VIRTUAL SUPPORT GROUP THAT WELCOMED INDIVIDUALS FROM ALL BACKGROUNDS, PROVIDING A SAFE SPACE FOR

THEM TO SHARE THEIR STRUGGLES, FEARS, AND ANXIETIES.

PARTICIPANTS IN MARK'S SUPPORT GROUP FOUND SOLACE IN KNOWING THAT THEY WERE NOT ALONE IN THEIR EXPERIENCES. THROUGH REGULAR VIDEO CALLS, THEY OFFERED EACH OTHER EMPATHY, UNDERSTANDING, AND PRACTICAL ADVICE ON COPING MECHANISMS. THE GROUP BECAME A LIFELINE FOR MANY, FOSTERING A SENSE OF CONNECTION AND REMINDING THEM OF THE POWER OF HUMAN CONNECTION, EVEN IN THE MIDST OF PHYSICAL DISTANCING.

MARK'S SUPPORT GROUP EXPANDED BEYOND THE VIRTUAL MEETINGS. PARTICIPANTS

ORGANIZED CARE PACKAGE EXCHANGES, ONLINE WELLNESS WORKSHOPS, AND EVEN VIRTUAL GAME NIGHTS TO UPLIFT SPIRITS AND MAINTAIN A SENSE OF COMMUNITY. THROUGH THEIR COLLECTIVE STRENGTH, THEY REMINDED ONE ANOTHER OF THE IMPORTANCE OF SELF-CARE, RESILIENCE, AND THE ENDURING POWER OF HUMAN KINDNESS.

SARAH'S NEIGHBORHOOD SUPPORT:

SARAH, A RESIDENT IN A TIGHT-KNIT NEIGHBORHOOD, WITNESSED THE CHALLENGES FACED BY HER NEIGHBORS DURING THE PANDEMIC. SHE TOOK IT UPON HERSELF TO CREATE A SUPPORT NETWORK WITHIN THE

COMMUNITY, OFFERING ASSISTANCE TO THOSE IN NEED.

WHETHER IT WAS GROCERY SHOPPING FOR ELDERLY NEIGHBORS, ORGANIZING VIRTUAL BOOK CLUBS FOR CHILDREN, OR PROVIDING EMOTIONAL SUPPORT TO STRUGGLING FAMILIES, SARAH BECAME THE GO-TO PERSON FOR HELP AND SUPPORT. HER GENUINE CARE AND WILLINGNESS TO LEND A HELPING HAND INSPIRED OTHERS TO JOIN HER CAUSE.

SOON, A WAVE OF SUPPORT SPREAD THROUGHOUT THE NEIGHBORHOOD. NEIGHBORS CHECKED IN ON EACH OTHER, SHARED RESOURCES, AND PROVIDED EMOTIONAL SUPPORT DURING TIMES OF

ISOLATION AND UNCERTAINTY. WHAT STARTED AS A SMALL ACT OF KINDNESS BY SARAH TRANSFORMED INTO A POWERFUL NETWORK OF COMPASSION AND MUTUAL AID THAT UPLIFTED THE ENTIRE COMMUNITY.

THESE STORIES HIGHLIGHT THE RESILIENCE, COMPASSION, AND ABILITY OF INDIVIDUALS TO SUPPORT EACH OTHER IN DIFFICULT TIMES. THROUGH THEIR STRENGTH AND ACTS OF KINDNESS, EMMA, MARK, SARAH, AND COUNTLESS OTHERS REMIND US THAT IN THE FACE OF ADVERSITY, WE CAN FIND STRENGTH WITHIN OURSELVES AND IN THE CONNECTIONS WE FORGE WITH ONE ANOTHER. THEIR STORIES SERVE AS A TESTAMENT TO THE INDOMITABLE HUMAN SPIRIT AND THE CAPACITY FOR

COMPASSION AND SUPPORT EVEN IN THE MOST CHALLENGING OF CIRCUMSTANCES.

FINANCIAL STRAINS AND MONEY MANAGEMENT

THE EMOTIONAL STRESS CAUSED BY FINANCIAL STRAINS, ESPECIALLY THE FEAR OF NOT BEING ABLE TO PROVIDE FOR LOVED ONES, CAN BE OVERWHELMING AND DEEPLY IMPACTFUL. THE WEIGHT OF FINANCIAL UNCERTAINTY CAN TAKE A TOLL ON INDIVIDUALS' MENTAL WELL-BEING AND CREATE A SENSE OF HELPLESSNESS. IT IS ESSENTIAL TO ADDRESS AND ACKNOWLEDGE THESE EMOTIONAL STRUGGLES, AS THEY ARE A COMMON EXPERIENCE FOR MANY DURING CHALLENGING TIMES.

1. **FEAR AND ANXIETY:** THE FEAR OF NOT BEING ABLE TO MEET FINANCIAL OBLIGATIONS AND PROVIDE FOR THE NEEDS OF LOVED ONES CAN TRIGGER INTENSE ANXIETY. THE CONSTANT

WORRY ABOUT JOB SECURITY, MOUNTING DEBTS, AND THE ABILITY TO COVER BASIC EXPENSES CAN CREATE A PERSISTENT STATE OF STRESS. THE FEAR OF LOSING ONE'S HOME, NOT HAVING ENOUGH TO PUT FOOD ON THE TABLE, OR BEING UNABLE TO AFFORD HEALTHCARE CAN LEAD TO A SENSE OF POWERLESSNESS AND DESPAIR.

2. **GUILT AND SHAME:** FINANCIAL STRAIN CAN EVOKE FEELINGS OF GUILT AND SHAME, AS INDIVIDUALS MAY PERCEIVE THEMSELVES AS FAILURES OR INADEQUATE FOR NOT BEING ABLE TO PROVIDE FOR THEIR LOVED ONES. THEY MAY INTERNALIZE THE SOCIETAL

PRESSURE TO BE FINANCIALLY SUCCESSFUL AND FEEL A SENSE OF SHAME FOR FALLING SHORT OF THOSE EXPECTATIONS. THIS EMOTIONAL BURDEN CAN BE ISOLATING, MAKING IT DIFFICULT FOR INDIVIDUALS TO SEEK HELP OR OPENLY DISCUSS THEIR STRUGGLES.

3. **IMPACT ON RELATIONSHIPS:**

FINANCIAL STRAIN CAN STRAIN RELATIONSHIPS, CAUSING TENSION AND CONFLICT WITHIN FAMILIES AND AMONG PARTNERS. THE PRESSURE TO MAKE ENDS MEET CAN LEAD TO STRAINED COMMUNICATION, ARGUMENTS OVER MONEY MATTERS, AND A SENSE OF DISCONNECTION. ADDITIONALLY,

INDIVIDUALS MAY FEEL A SENSE OF GUILT OR RESPONSIBILITY FOR NOT BEING ABLE TO FULFILL THEIR LOVED ONES' DESIRES OR NEEDS, WHICH CAN FURTHER STRAIN RELATIONSHIPS AND IMPACT EMOTIONAL WELL-BEING.

4. **SELF-WORTH AND IDENTITY:** FINANCIAL STRUGGLES CAN CHALLENGE AN INDIVIDUAL'S SENSE OF SELF-WORTH AND IDENTITY, AS SOCIETAL NORMS OFTEN EQUATE FINANCIAL SUCCESS WITH PERSONAL VALUE. THE INABILITY TO MAINTAIN A CERTAIN STANDARD OF LIVING OR ACHIEVE FINANCIAL GOALS MAY LEAD TO FEELINGS OF INADEQUACY AND A LOSS OF SELF-ESTEEM. IT IS

IMPORTANT TO REMEMBER THAT FINANCIAL CIRCUMSTANCES DO NOT DEFINE A PERSON'S WORTH, BUT THE EMOTIONAL TOLL OF SOCIETAL EXPECTATIONS CAN BE SIGNIFICANT.

ADDRESSING THE EMOTIONAL STRESS CAUSED BY FINANCIAL STRAINS REQUIRES COMPASSION, SUPPORT, AND UNDERSTANDING. HERE ARE A FEW SUGGESTIONS:

1. **SEEK SUPPORT:** REACH OUT TO TRUSTED FRIENDS, FAMILY MEMBERS, OR SUPPORT GROUPS TO SHARE YOUR FEELINGS AND CONCERNS. IT CAN BE HELPFUL TO TALK OPENLY ABOUT YOUR FINANCIAL STRESS AND RECEIVE EMPATHY

AND ENCOURAGEMENT FROM OTHERS WHO MAY HAVE EXPERIENCED SIMILAR CHALLENGES.

2. **PRACTICE SELF-CARE:** TAKE CARE OF YOUR MENTAL AND EMOTIONAL WELL-BEING BY ENGAGING IN ACTIVITIES THAT BRING YOU JOY AND RELAXATION. PRACTICE MINDFULNESS, ENGAGE IN PHYSICAL EXERCISE, OR PURSUE HOBBIES THAT PROVIDE A SENSE OF FULFILLMENT. PRIORITIZING SELF-CARE CAN HELP ALLEVIATE STRESS AND IMPROVE OVERALL RESILIENCE.

3. **SEEK FINANCIAL GUIDANCE:** CONSIDER REACHING OUT TO FINANCIAL PROFESSIONALS OR COUNSELORS WHO

CAN PROVIDE GUIDANCE ON MANAGING YOUR FINANCES, CREATING BUDGETS, AND EXPLORING OPTIONS FOR DEBT MANAGEMENT. TAKING PROACTIVE STEPS TOWARDS IMPROVING YOUR FINANCIAL SITUATION CAN ALLEVIATE SOME OF THE EMOTIONAL STRESS ASSOCIATED WITH FINANCIAL STRAIN.

4. **ADJUST EXPECTATIONS:** RECOGNIZE THAT FINANCIAL DIFFICULTIES ARE OFTEN TEMPORARY AND THAT EVERYONE FACES SETBACKS AT SOME POINT IN THEIR LIVES. ADJUST YOUR EXPECTATIONS AND FOCUS ON BUILDING RESILIENCE AND SEEKING SOLUTIONS RATHER THAN FIXATING ON PERCEIVED FAILURES.

5. **COMMUNICATE WITH LOVED ONES:** OPENLY COMMUNICATE WITH YOUR LOVED ONES ABOUT YOUR FINANCIAL SITUATION AND COLLABORATE ON FINDING WAYS TO NAVIGATE THE CHALLENGES TOGETHER. SHARING YOUR FEARS AND CONCERNS CAN FOSTER A SENSE OF UNDERSTANDING AND UNITY, STRENGTHENING RELATIONSHIPS IN THE FACE OF ADVERSITY.

REMEMBER, YOU ARE NOT ALONE IN YOUR FINANCIAL STRUGGLES, AND THERE IS SUPPORT AVAILABLE. BY ADDRESSING THE EMOTIONAL STRESS CAUSED BY FINANCIAL STRAINS AND

SEEKING ASSISTANCE WHEN NEEDED, YOU CAN NAVIGATE THESE CHALLENGES WITH RESILIENCE AND FIND A SENSE OF HOPE FOR THE FUTURE.

DURING CHALLENGING TIMES OF FINANCIAL STRAIN, IT'S IMPORTANT TO SEEK PRACTICAL GUIDANCE AND UTILIZE AVAILABLE RESOURCES THAT CAN OFFER HOPE AND REASSURANCE. HERE ARE SOME PRACTICAL STEPS AND RESOURCES TO CONSIDER:

1. **CREATE A BUDGET:** DEVELOPING A BUDGET HELPS YOU GAIN A CLEAR UNDERSTANDING OF YOUR INCOME AND EXPENSES. START BY LISTING YOUR

MONTHLY INCOME AND TRACKING YOUR EXPENSES. IDENTIFY AREAS WHERE YOU CAN REDUCE UNNECESSARY SPENDING AND PRIORITIZE ESSENTIAL NEEDS. BUDGETING TOOLS AND APPS, SUCH AS MINT AND YOU NEED A BUDGET (YNAB), CAN ASSIST YOU IN MANAGING YOUR FINANCES EFFECTIVELY.

2. **EXPLORE FINANCIAL ASSISTANCE PROGRAMS:** RESEARCH AND EXPLORE AVAILABLE FINANCIAL ASSISTANCE PROGRAMS IN YOUR LOCAL COMMUNITY OR COUNTRY. GOVERNMENTS, NON-PROFIT ORGANIZATIONS, AND CHARITABLE FOUNDATIONS OFTEN PROVIDE ASSISTANCE FOR HOUSING,

FOOD, UTILITIES, AND OTHER ESSENTIAL NEEDS DURING DIFFICULT TIMES. REACH OUT TO LOCAL SOCIAL SERVICES AGENCIES OR VISIT THEIR WEBSITES FOR INFORMATION ON ELIGIBILITY AND APPLICATION PROCESSES.

3. **SEEK EMPLOYMENT AND CAREER SUPPORT:** IF YOU ARE EXPERIENCING JOB LOSS OR STRUGGLING TO FIND EMPLOYMENT, UTILIZE CAREER SUPPORT SERVICES PROVIDED BY GOVERNMENT AGENCIES OR CAREER CENTERS. THEY CAN ASSIST YOU WITH JOB SEARCH STRATEGIES, RESUME WRITING, INTERVIEW PREPARATION, AND CONNECTING WITH POTENTIAL

EMPLOYERS. ONLINE JOB PLATFORMS AND PROFESSIONAL NETWORKING SITES LIKE LINKEDIN CAN ALSO HELP IN EXPLORING NEW JOB OPPORTUNITIES.

4. **CONSIDER FINANCIAL COUNSELING:** FINANCIAL COUNSELING SERVICES CAN PROVIDE EXPERT GUIDANCE AND ADVICE TAILORED TO YOUR SPECIFIC FINANCIAL SITUATION. COUNSELORS CAN HELP YOU CREATE A PLAN TO MANAGE DEBT, NEGOTIATE WITH CREDITORS, AND DEVELOP LONG-TERM FINANCIAL GOALS. NON-PROFIT ORGANIZATIONS, CREDIT COUNSELING AGENCIES, AND FINANCIAL PLANNERS CAN OFFER ASSISTANCE IN THIS AREA.

5. **EXPLORE COMMUNITY RESOURCES:** MANY COMMUNITIES HAVE LOCAL INITIATIVES AND ORGANIZATIONS THAT OFFER SUPPORT DURING FINANCIAL HARDSHIPS. THESE RESOURCES CAN INCLUDE FOOD BANKS, COMMUNITY KITCHENS, FREE OR LOW-COST MEDICAL CLINICS, AND SUPPORT GROUPS. REACH OUT TO COMMUNITY CENTERS, RELIGIOUS INSTITUTIONS, OR LOCAL SOCIAL SERVICE AGENCIES TO LEARN ABOUT AVAILABLE RESOURCES IN YOUR AREA.

6. **PRIORITIZE MENTAL HEALTH AND WELL-BEING:** THE EMOTIONAL TOLL OF

FINANCIAL STRAIN CAN BE SIGNIFICANT, IMPACTING OVERALL WELL-BEING. TAKE CARE OF YOUR MENTAL HEALTH BY SEEKING SUPPORT FROM MENTAL HEALTH PROFESSIONALS, JOINING SUPPORT GROUPS, PRACTICING SELF-CARE ACTIVITIES, AND ENGAGING IN STRESS-REDUCING PRACTICES SUCH AS MEDITATION OR EXERCISE. ONLINE PLATFORMS LIKE BETTERHELP AND TALKSPACE OFFER ACCESSIBLE COUNSELING SERVICES.

7. **EDUCATE YOURSELF:** TAKE ADVANTAGE OF FREE FINANCIAL EDUCATION RESOURCES AVAILABLE ONLINE OR THROUGH LOCAL

COMMUNITY ORGANIZATIONS. THESE RESOURCES CAN PROVIDE INFORMATION ON BUDGETING, DEBT MANAGEMENT, INVESTING, AND BUILDING FINANCIAL RESILIENCE. ONLINE COURSES, PODCASTS, AND BLOGS FROM REPUTABLE FINANCIAL EXPERTS CAN OFFER VALUABLE INSIGHTS AND STRATEGIES.

8. **MAINTAIN OPEN COMMUNICATION:** KEEP OPEN LINES OF COMMUNICATION WITH YOUR LOVED ONES ABOUT YOUR FINANCIAL SITUATION. DISCUSSING CHALLENGES AND BRAINSTORMING SOLUTIONS TOGETHER CAN PROVIDE EMOTIONAL SUPPORT AND HELP ALLEVIATE THE BURDEN. CONSIDER

SEEKING PROFESSIONAL RELATIONSHIP COUNSELING IF FINANCIAL STRAINS ARE IMPACTING YOUR RELATIONSHIPS SIGNIFICANTLY.

REMEMBER, EVERYONE'S FINANCIAL SITUATION IS UNIQUE, AND FINDING THE RIGHT SOLUTIONS MAY TAKE TIME AND PERSISTENCE. UTILIZE THESE PRACTICAL STEPS AND RESOURCES TO EMPOWER YOURSELF, SEEK GUIDANCE, AND FIND HOPE DURING TIMES OF FINANCIAL STRAIN. WITH DETERMINATION, SUPPORT, AND A PROACTIVE APPROACH, YOU CAN NAVIGATE THROUGH THESE CHALLENGES AND WORK TOWARDS A MORE STABLE AND HOPEFUL FINANCIAL FUTURE.

CRISES IN FOOD, HEALTH, AND WATER

THE COMMUNITY FOOD BANK:

IN A SMALL TOWN HIT HARD BY THE PANDEMIC, THE LOCAL COMMUNITY CAME TOGETHER TO ESTABLISH A FOOD BANK. PEOPLE FROM ALL WALKS OF LIFE VOLUNTEERED THEIR TIME AND RESOURCES TO COLLECT AND DISTRIBUTE FOOD

TO THOSE IN NEED. FAMILIES STRUGGLING WITH FOOD INSECURITY FOUND SOLACE IN THE KINDNESS AND COMPASSION SHOWN BY THEIR NEIGHBORS. DONATIONS POURED IN FROM LOCAL BUSINESSES, SCHOOLS, AND INDIVIDUALS, ENSURING THAT NO ONE WENT HUNGRY. THE FOOD BANK BECAME A SYMBOL OF HOPE AND UNITY, DEMONSTRATING THE POWER OF COMMUNITY SUPPORT IN ALLEVIATING THE CRISIS OF FOOD INSECURITY.

THE MOBILE HEALTHCARE CLINIC:

RECOGNIZING THE LACK OF ACCESS TO HEALTHCARE IN UNDERSERVED COMMUNITIES, A GROUP OF MEDICAL PROFESSIONALS AND VOLUNTEERS TOOK ACTION. THEY

TRANSFORMED AN OLD BUS INTO A MOBILE HEALTHCARE CLINIC THAT TRAVELED TO REMOTE AREAS, OFFERING FREE MEDICAL SERVICES AND SCREENINGS. WITH A FOCUS ON PREVENTIVE CARE, THEY EDUCATED INDIVIDUALS AND FAMILIES ABOUT HEALTHY LIVING, DISTRIBUTED ESSENTIAL MEDICATIONS, AND PROVIDED MUCH-NEEDED CHECK-UPS. THIS INITIATIVE NOT ONLY ADDRESSED IMMEDIATE HEALTH CONCERNS BUT ALSO INSTILLED HOPE AND A SENSE OF BELONGING IN THOSE WHO HAD BEEN NEGLECTED BY THE TRADITIONAL HEALTHCARE SYSTEM.

THE CLEAN WATER INITIATIVE:

IN A VILLAGE PLAGUED BY CONTAMINATED WATER SOURCES, A TEAM OF ENGINEERS, ENVIRONMENTALISTS, AND DEDICATED VOLUNTEERS EMBARKED ON A MISSION TO PROVIDE CLEAN WATER TO THE COMMUNITY. THEY INSTALLED WATER FILTRATION SYSTEMS, REPAIRED WELLS, AND IMPLEMENTED WATER MANAGEMENT PRACTICES TO ENSURE A SUSTAINABLE SUPPLY OF SAFE DRINKING WATER. THE IMPACT WAS TRANSFORMATIVE, AS FAMILIES NO LONGER HAD TO WORRY ABOUT WATERBORNE DISEASES AND CHILDREN COULD FOCUS ON THEIR EDUCATION INSTEAD OF SPENDING HOURS FETCHING WATER. THIS INITIATIVE SPARKED A RENEWED SENSE OF HOPE

AND IMPROVED THE OVERALL WELL-BEING OF
THE ENTIRE COMMUNITY.

THESE STORIES HIGHLIGHT THE INCREDIBLE
ACTS OF COMPASSION AND THE POWER OF
COMMUNITY SUPPORT IN TIMES OF CRISES.
THEY SHOWCASE HOW INDIVIDUALS AND
ORGANIZATIONS CAN COME TOGETHER TO
ALLEVIATE THE HARDSHIPS FACED BY THOSE
STRUGGLING WITH FOOD INSECURITY, LACK OF
HEALTHCARE ACCESS, AND CLEAN WATER.
THROUGH COLLECTIVE EFFORTS, EMPATHY, AND
A COMMITMENT TO MAKING A DIFFERENCE,
THESE INITIATIVES DEMONSTRATE THAT
POSITIVE CHANGE IS POSSIBLE, EVEN IN THE
FACE OF OVERWHELMING CHALLENGES. THEY
INSPIRE US TO TAKE ACTION, SUPPORT ONE

ANOTHER, AND WORK TOWARDS BUILDING A MORE COMPASSIONATE AND RESILIENT WORLD.

EMILY'S FOOD INSECURITY:

EMILY, A SINGLE MOTHER OF TWO, FOUND HERSELF FACING THE HARSH REALITY OF FOOD INSECURITY DURING THE PANDEMIC. WITH HER HOURS AT WORK REDUCED AND HER INCOME DIMINISHED, SHE STRUGGLED TO PROVIDE NUTRITIOUS MEALS FOR HER CHILDREN. EMILY OFTEN WENT TO BED WITH A GNAWING FEELING IN HER STOMACH, WORRIED ABOUT HER KIDS GOING TO BED HUNGRY.

EVERY DAY, EMILY WOULD WALK PAST THE LOCAL GROCERY STORE, LONGING TO FILL HER

SHOPPING CART WITH FRESH PRODUCE AND WHOLESOME INGREDIENTS. BUT THE RISING COST OF FOOD MADE IT INCREASINGLY DIFFICULT FOR HER TO MAKE ENDS MEET. SHE COULDN'T BEAR TO SEE HER CHILDREN'S DISAPPOINTED FACES AS THEY OPENED AN ALMOST EMPTY FRIDGE.

HOWEVER, IN THE MIDST OF HER DESPAIR, EMILY DISCOVERED A LOCAL FOOD PANTRY THAT PROVIDED ESSENTIAL GROCERIES TO FAMILIES IN NEED. WITH TEARS STREAMING DOWN HER FACE, SHE GRATEFULLY ACCEPTED THE FRESH VEGETABLES, CANNED GOODS, AND OTHER SUPPLIES THAT WOULD SUSTAIN HER FAMILY FOR THE WEEK. THE KINDNESS AND SUPPORT FROM THE VOLUNTEERS AT THE FOOD

PANTRY BROUGHT A GLIMMER OF HOPE BACK INTO EMILY'S LIFE, REMINDING HER THAT SHE WAS NOT ALONE IN HER STRUGGLE.

JAVIER'S LACK OF HEALTHCARE ACCESS:

JAVIER, A HARDWORKING FATHER, FACED A CHALLENGING DILEMMA DURING THE PANDEMIC. HE EXPERIENCED CONCERNING SYMPTOMS BUT COULDN'T AFFORD TO SEEK MEDICAL ATTENTION. AS THE SOLE BREADWINNER FOR HIS FAMILY, HE HAD TO PRIORITIZE PUTTING FOOD ON THE TABLE AND PAYING BILLS OVER HIS OWN HEALTH.

DAYS TURNED INTO WEEKS, AND JAVIER'S SYMPTOMS WORSENED. HE LIVED WITH CONSTANT FEAR, NOT ONLY FOR HIMSELF BUT ALSO FOR THE WELL-BEING OF HIS FAMILY. THE LACK OF ACCESS TO AFFORDABLE HEALTHCARE LEFT HIM FEELING HELPLESS AND VULNERABLE.

FORTUNATELY, JAVIER DISCOVERED A COMMUNITY CLINIC THAT PROVIDED FREE OR LOW-COST HEALTHCARE SERVICES TO UNINSURED INDIVIDUALS. WITH A MIX OF RELIEF AND TREPIDATION, HE MADE AN APPOINTMENT AND FINALLY RECEIVED THE MEDICAL CARE HE DESPERATELY NEEDED. THE DEDICATED HEALTHCARE PROFESSIONALS NOT ONLY ADDRESSED HIS IMMEDIATE CONCERNS BUT ALSO CONNECTED HIM WITH RESOURCES

FOR ONGOING SUPPORT AND AFFORDABLE MEDICATIONS.

MAYA'S STRUGGLE FOR CLEAN WATER:

MAYA LIVED IN A RURAL VILLAGE WHERE ACCESS TO CLEAN WATER WAS A CONSTANT STRUGGLE, EXACERBATED BY THE PANDEMIC. THE UNRELIABLE WATER SUPPLY AND LACK OF PROPER SANITATION FACILITIES POSED A SIGNIFICANT THREAT TO THE HEALTH AND WELL-BEING OF THE COMMUNITY, ESPECIALLY DURING A TIME WHEN PROPER HYGIENE WAS CRUCIAL.

MAYA SPENT HOURS EACH DAY TREKKING TO DISTANT WATER SOURCES, CARRYING HEAVY CONTAINERS ON HER BACK, JUST TO ENSURE

HER FAMILY HAD ENOUGH WATER FOR DRINKING, COOKING, AND CLEANING. THE BURDEN OF THIS DAILY TASK TOOK A TOLL ON HER PHYSICAL AND EMOTIONAL WELL-BEING. SHE DREAMED OF A DAY WHEN CLEAN WATER WOULD FLOW FREELY FROM TAPS IN HER VILLAGE, RELIEVING HER AND HER NEIGHBORS FROM THE CONSTANT WORRY OF WATERBORNE DISEASES.

IN THE FACE OF THESE CHALLENGES, MAYA JOINED FORCES WITH COMMUNITY MEMBERS AND LOCAL ORGANIZATIONS TO ADVOCATE FOR CLEAN WATER INITIATIVES. THROUGH THEIR COLLECTIVE EFFORTS, THEY RAISED AWARENESS, SECURED FUNDING, AND IMPLEMENTED PROJECTS THAT IMPROVED ACCESS TO CLEAN

WATER AND SANITATION FACILITIES IN THEIR VILLAGE. MAYA'S DETERMINATION AND THE UNWAVERING SUPPORT OF HER COMMUNITY TRANSFORMED THEIR LIVES, BRINGING HOPE, HEALTH, AND A BRIGHTER FUTURE.

THESE STORIES OF INDIVIDUALS STRUGGLING WITH FOOD INSECURITY, LACK OF HEALTHCARE ACCESS, AND CLEAN WATER EVOKE EMPATHY AND REMIND US OF THE PROFOUND IMPACT THESE CHALLENGES HAVE ON PEOPLE'S LIVES. THEY HIGHLIGHT THE URGENT NEED FOR COLLECTIVE ACTION, COMPASSION, AND SUPPORT TO ADDRESS THESE FUNDAMENTAL ISSUES AND ENSURE THAT EVERYONE HAS ACCESS TO THE BASIC NECESSITIES FOR A DIGNIFIED LIFE. BY SHARING THESE EMOTIONAL

STORIES, WE CAN FOSTER EMPATHY, INSPIRE ACTION, AND WORK TOWARDS A MORE JUST AND EQUITABLE WORLD.

STORIES OF RESILIENCE AND SURVIVAL

DURING THE PANDEMIC, NUMEROUS ACTS OF KINDNESS, SELFLESSNESS, AND UNITY HAVE EMERGED, UPLIFTING THE HUMAN SPIRIT AND REMINDING US OF THE POWER OF COMPASSION. HERE ARE A FEW EXAMPLES:

1. **NEIGHBORHOOD SUPPORT NETWORKS:** IN COMMUNITIES AROUND THE WORLD, NEIGHBORS RALLIED TOGETHER TO CREATE SUPPORT NETWORKS. THEY ORGANIZED GROCERY

SHOPPING TRIPS FOR THE ELDERLY AND VULNERABLE, SHARED ESSENTIAL SUPPLIES, AND OFFERED EMOTIONAL SUPPORT. THIS GRASSROOTS MOVEMENT SHOWCASED THE STRENGTH OF UNITY AND THE WILLINGNESS OF PEOPLE TO LEND A HELPING HAND.

2. **HEALTHCARE HEROES:** HEALTHCARE PROFESSIONALS BECAME THE TRUE HEROES OF THE PANDEMIC, RISKING THEIR LIVES AND WORKING TIRELESSLY TO SAVE OTHERS. THEIR SELFLESSNESS AND UNWAVERING DEDICATION INSPIRED ADMIRATION AND GRATITUDE FROM PEOPLE WORLDWIDE. FROM DOCTORS AND NURSES TO JANITORS AND ADMINISTRATIVE STAFF, THESE FRONTLINE WORKERS DISPLAYED IMMENSE COURAGE, COMPASSION, AND RESILIENCE.

3. **MUTUAL AID GROUPS:** MUTUAL AID GROUPS SPRANG UP GLOBALLY, CONNECTING VOLUNTEERS WITH THOSE IN NEED. THESE GROUPS PROVIDED PRACTICAL SUPPORT, SUCH AS DELIVERING GROCERIES AND MEDICATION TO INDIVIDUALS IN QUARANTINE, OFFERING VIRTUAL MENTAL HEALTH COUNSELING, AND COORDINATING RESOURCES FOR VULNERABLE POPULATIONS. THEY DEMONSTRATED THE POWER OF COMMUNITY-DRIVEN INITIATIVES AND THE INCREDIBLE IMPACT OF COLLECTIVE EFFORTS.

4. **DONATIONS AND PHILANTHROPY:** IN THE FACE OF ECONOMIC UNCERTAINTY, MANY INDIVIDUALS, CELEBRITIES, AND CORPORATIONS STEPPED FORWARD WITH GENEROUS DONATIONS. THEY

CONTRIBUTED FUNDS TO SUPPORT MEDICAL RESEARCH, PROVIDED GRANTS FOR STRUGGLING SMALL BUSINESSES, AND FUNDED INITIATIVES TO ADDRESS FOOD INSECURITY AND HOMELESSNESS. THESE ACTS OF GENEROSITY HIGHLIGHTED THE IMPORTANCE OF STANDING TOGETHER AND HELPING THOSE WHO ARE MOST IN NEED.

5. **CREATIVE INITIATIVES:** ARTISTS, MUSICIANS, AND PERFORMERS FOUND INNOVATIVE WAYS TO UPLIFT SPIRITS AND FOSTER A SENSE OF TOGETHERNESS. ONLINE CONCERTS, VIRTUAL ART EXHIBITIONS, AND LIVE-STREAMED PERFORMANCES BROUGHT JOY AND INSPIRATION TO PEOPLE'S LIVES. THESE CREATIVE INITIATIVES REMINDED US OF THE TRANSFORMATIVE POWER OF ART AND ITS ABILITY TO UNITE AND HEAL.

6. **SOLIDARITY AND SUPPORT FOR MARGINALIZED COMMUNITIES:** THE PANDEMIC UNDERSCORED EXISTING INEQUALITIES, WITH MARGINALIZED COMMUNITIES DISPROPORTIONATELY AFFECTED. HOWEVER, INDIVIDUALS AND ORGANIZATIONS RALLIED TO SUPPORT THESE COMMUNITIES. THEY PROVIDED ESSENTIAL RESOURCES, ADVOCATED FOR THEIR RIGHTS, AND RAISED AWARENESS ABOUT SYSTEMIC INJUSTICES. THE OUTPOURING OF SUPPORT DEMONSTRATED A COMMITMENT TO INCLUSIVITY, EQUITY, AND JUSTICE.

THESE ACTS OF KINDNESS, SELFLESSNESS, AND UNITY REMIND US THAT EVEN IN THE DARKEST OF TIMES, THE HUMAN SPIRIT SHINES BRIGHT. THEY INSPIRE US TO LOOK BEYOND OURSELVES, TO EXTEND A HELPING HAND, AND TO FOSTER A SENSE OF UNITY AND COMPASSION. THEY SERVE

AS A POWERFUL TESTAMENT TO THE RESILIENCE AND EMPATHY INHERENT WITHIN US ALL.

EMMA'S JOURNEY OF RESILIENCE:

EMMA, A YOUNG WOMAN WITH A PHYSICAL DISABILITY, FACED NUMEROUS OBSTACLES THROUGHOUT HER LIFE. DESPITE THE CHALLENGES, SHE REFUSED TO LET HER CIRCUMSTANCES DEFINE HER. EMMA'S DETERMINATION AND POSITIVE MINDSET BECAME HER DRIVING FORCE. SHE WORKED HARD TO ACHIEVE HER GOALS, PURSUING HIGHER EDUCATION AND ADVOCATING FOR DISABILITY RIGHTS.

THROUGH HER RESILIENCE, EMMA BECAME AN INSPIRATION TO OTHERS. SHE SHARED HER STORY OF TRIUMPH OVER ADVERSITY, EMPOWERING INDIVIDUALS FACING SIMILAR CHALLENGES TO BELIEVE IN THEIR OWN ABILITIES. EMMA'S UNWAVERING SPIRIT AND UNWAVERING BELIEF IN HERSELF SERVED AS A REMINDER THAT ONE'S LIMITATIONS DO NOT HAVE TO DEFINE THEIR POTENTIAL.

MICHAEL'S JOURNEY FROM HOMELESSNESS TO SUCCESS:

MICHAEL FOUND HIMSELF HOMELESS AFTER LOSING HIS JOB AND FACING FINANCIAL DIFFICULTIES. HE WAS LIVING ON THE STREETS, STRUGGLING TO SURVIVE. HOWEVER, HE

REFUSED TO GIVE UP ON HIMSELF. MICHAEL ENROLLED IN A LOCAL JOB TRAINING PROGRAM, DETERMINED TO TURN HIS LIFE AROUND.

WITH PERSEVERANCE AND HARD WORK, MICHAEL SECURED EMPLOYMENT AND GRADUALLY IMPROVED HIS SITUATION. HE SAVED MONEY, OBTAINED STABLE HOUSING, AND REBUILT HIS LIFE. INSPIRED BY HIS EXPERIENCE, MICHAEL BECAME AN ADVOCATE FOR HOMELESS INDIVIDUALS, SHARING HIS STORY TO RAISE AWARENESS AND SUPPORT FOR THOSE FACING SIMILAR CHALLENGES. HIS JOURNEY SHOWCASED THE POWER OF RESILIENCE AND THE POTENTIAL FOR TRANSFORMATION EVEN IN THE MOST CHALLENGING CIRCUMSTANCES.

SOPHIA'S JOURNEY OF HEALING AND FORGIVENESS:

SOPHIA ENDURED A TRAUMATIC EXPERIENCE THAT LEFT HER EMOTIONALLY SCARRED. HOWEVER, INSTEAD OF ALLOWING ANGER AND RESENTMENT TO CONSUME HER, SHE EMBARKED ON A JOURNEY OF HEALING AND FORGIVENESS. THROUGH THERAPY, SELF-REFLECTION, AND SUPPORT FROM LOVED ONES, SOPHIA FOUND THE STRENGTH TO LET GO OF THE PAIN AND EMBRACE A PATH OF HEALING.

AS SHE EMBRACED FORGIVENESS, SOPHIA DISCOVERED A NEWFOUND SENSE OF FREEDOM AND INNER PEACE. SHE STARTED SHARING HER STORY, SPREADING A MESSAGE OF HEALING,

COMPASSION, AND THE POWER OF FORGIVENESS. SOPHIA'S STORY TOUCHED THE HEARTS OF MANY, INSPIRING OTHERS TO EMBARK ON THEIR OWN JOURNEYS OF HEALING AND FORGIVENESS, REMINDING THEM THAT IT IS POSSIBLE TO FIND LIGHT EVEN IN THE DARKEST OF TIMES.

THESE STORIES OF TRIUMPH OVER ADVERSITY HIGHLIGHT THE INDOMITABLE HUMAN SPIRIT AND THE POWER OF RESILIENCE, DETERMINATION, AND FORGIVENESS. THEY REMIND US THAT NO MATTER THE CHALLENGES WE FACE, WE HAVE THE ABILITY TO OVERCOME AND CREATE A BETTER FUTURE FOR OURSELVES AND OTHERS. THESE INSPIRING INDIVIDUALS SERVE AS BEACONS OF HOPE, DEMONSTRATING

THAT EVEN IN THE FACE OF ADVERSITY, THERE

IS ALWAYS A PATH TO TRIUMPH.

CONCLUSION

THROUGHOUT THE PAGES OF THE EBOOK, THE EMOTIONAL JOURNEY OF THE COMMON MAN IN THE FACE OF THE COVID-19 PANDEMIC UNFOLDS WITH DEPTH AND COMPLEXITY. IT IS A JOURNEY MARKED BY HARDSHIP, LOSS, AND UNCERTAINTY, BUT ALSO BY RESILIENCE, STRENGTH, AND THE UNWAVERING HUMAN SPIRIT.

FROM THE STRUGGLES OF FAMILIES GRAPPLING WITH JOB LOSS, REMOTE LEARNING, AND HEALTH CONCERNS TO THE EMOTIONAL TOLL ON STUDENTS, THE CHALLENGES FACED BY ENTREPRENEURS AND WORKERS, AND THE IMPACT ON THE WORLD OF CINEMA, SPORTS, AND THE ARTS, THE EBOOK DELVES INTO THE MULTIFACETED ASPECTS OF THE PANDEMIC'S IMPACT ON INDIVIDUALS AND COMMUNITIES.

THE STORIES SHARED WITHIN THE EBOOK EVOKE A RANGE OF EMOTIONS - FEAR, ANXIETY, SADNESS, FRUSTRATION, AND DESPAIR. THEY REFLECT THE COLLECTIVE GRIEF EXPERIENCED ON A GLOBAL SCALE AS LIVES WERE UPENDED, DREAMS PUT ON HOLD, AND LOVED ONES LOST. THE EMOTIONAL TOLL IS PALPABLE, HIGHLIGHTING THE DEPTHS OF THE CHALLENGES FACED BY THE COMMON MAN.

HOWEVER, AMIDST THE DARKNESS, THERE IS A PREVAILING THEME OF RESILIENCE AND THE INDOMITABLE HUMAN SPIRIT. THE COMMON MAN, IN ALL THEIR DIVERSITY AND CIRCUMSTANCES, FINDS STRENGTH WITHIN THEMSELVES AND THEIR COMMUNITIES. THEY ADAPT, SUPPORT ONE ANOTHER, AND DISCOVER INNOVATIVE WAYS TO NAVIGATE THE ADVERSITIES.

THE EBOOK SHOWCASES INSPIRING STORIES OF FAMILIES WHO, DESPITE FACING FINANCIAL HARDSHIPS, SEPARATION, AND LOSS, FIND SOLACE IN THEIR BONDS, SUPPORTING AND LIFTING EACH OTHER UP. STUDENTS, DESPITE

FEELINGS OF ISOLATION, ANXIETY, AND
ACADEMIC CHALLENGES, DEMONSTRATE
REMARKABLE ADAPTABILITY AND A THIRST
FOR KNOWLEDGE.

ENTREPRENEURS AND WORKERS DISPLAY
UNWAVERING DETERMINATION, FINDING
INNOVATIVE SOLUTIONS, COLLABORATING
VIRTUALLY, AND SUPPORTING THEIR
COMMUNITIES. ARTISTS, FILMMAKERS,
ATHLETES, AND INDIVIDUALS FROM VARIOUS
FIELDS EXEMPLIFY CREATIVE RESILIENCE, USING
THEIR TALENTS TO UPLIFT AND HEAL.

THE EBOOK ALSO SHEDS LIGHT ON THE DEEP
EMPATHY AND COMPASSION THAT EMERGES
DURING CRISES. COMMUNITIES COME
TOGETHER TO ESTABLISH FOOD BANKS, MOBILE
HEALTHCARE CLINICS, AND INITIATIVES FOR
CLEAN WATER. INDIVIDUALS EXTEND HELPING
HANDS TO THEIR NEIGHBORS, PROVIDING
ESSENTIAL SUPPORT AND REMINDING US OF THE
POWER OF UNITY.

ULTIMATELY, THE EBOOK HIGHLIGHTS THE TRIUMPH OF THE COMMON MAN'S RESILIENCE. IT REMINDS US THAT EVEN IN THE FACE OF ADVERSITY, HUMANITY'S INNATE STRENGTH AND ABILITY TO ENDURE SHINE THROUGH. IT IS A TESTAMENT TO THE UNWAVERING SPIRIT THAT CARRIES INDIVIDUALS AND COMMUNITIES FORWARD, FORGING A PATH OF SURVIVAL AND EVENTUAL RECOVERY.

THROUGH THE EMOTIONAL JOURNEY PRESENTED IN THE EBOOK, READERS ARE INVITED TO WITNESS THE CHALLENGES, EMPATHIZE WITH THE STRUGGLES, AND ULTIMATELY CELEBRATE THE RESILIENCE OF THE COMMON MAN. IT IS A TESTAMENT TO THE HUMAN CAPACITY TO OVERCOME, REBUILD, AND FIND HOPE EVEN IN THE DARKEST OF TIMES.

IN THE MIDST OF THE TRIALS AND

TRIBULATIONS WE HAVE FACED, LET US HOLD

ONTO A MESSAGE OF HOPE, GRATITUDE, AND

THE ENDURING STRENGTH OF THE HUMAN HEART.

HOPE IS THE GUIDING LIGHT THAT PIERCES THROUGH THE DARKEST OF NIGHTS. IT REMINDS US THAT BETTER DAYS ARE AHEAD, AND THAT OUR COLLECTIVE RESILIENCE WILL CARRY US THROUGH. IT IS THE SPARK THAT IGNITES OUR DETERMINATION TO OVERCOME, TO REBUILD, AND TO CREATE A BRIGHTER FUTURE.

GRATITUDE IS THE FOUNDATION UPON WHICH WE CAN FIND SOLACE AND APPRECIATION FOR THE BLESSINGS THAT SURROUND US. IT IS THE RECOGNITION OF THE SMALL JOYS, THE ACTS OF KINDNESS, AND THE MOMENTS OF CONNECTION

THAT BRING WARMTH TO OUR HEARTS. LET US BE GRATEFUL FOR THE SUPPORT WE RECEIVE, FOR THE LOVE OF OUR FAMILIES AND FRIENDS, AND FOR THE COUNTLESS EVERYDAY HEROES WHO HAVE SELFLESSLY DEDICATED THEMSELVES TO HELPING OTHERS.

THE HUMAN HEART IS A WELLSPRING OF STRENGTH THAT BEATS WITHIN EACH AND EVERY ONE OF US. IT IS RESILIENT, COMPASSIONATE, AND FILLED WITH BOUNDLESS POTENTIAL. IT IS THIS STRENGTH THAT HAS CARRIED US THROUGH THE DARKEST HOURS, LIFTING US UP WHEN WE THOUGHT WE COULD NOT GO ON. IT IS A TESTAMENT TO OUR ABILITY TO ENDURE, TO ADAPT, AND TO FIND WITHIN

OURSELVES THE COURAGE TO FACE ANY
CHALLENGE.

IN OUR JOURNEY THROUGH THE PAGES OF THIS
EBOOK AND IN OUR OWN LIVES, LET US
REMEMBER THAT HOPE, GRATITUDE, AND THE
ENDURING STRENGTH OF THE HUMAN HEART
ARE THE GUIDING FORCES THAT WILL LEAD US
FORWARD. THEY REMIND US THAT WE ARE
NEVER ALONE, AND THAT TOGETHER WE CAN
CONQUER ANY OBSTACLE.

AS WE TURN THE FINAL PAGE, LET US HOLD
ONTO THESE TRUTHS. LET US EMBRACE HOPE AS
A BEACON OF LIGHT, GRATITUDE AS A SOURCE
OF COMFORT, AND THE STRENGTH OF OUR
HEARTS AS A REMINDER OF OUR LIMITLESS

POTENTIAL. WITH THESE PILLARS, WE CAN FACE THE FUTURE WITH COURAGE, COMPASSION, AND UNWAVERING DETERMINATION.

MAY OUR HEARTS BE FILLED WITH HOPE, MAY OUR SPIRITS BE UPLIFTED BY GRATITUDE, AND MAY WE ALWAYS FIND THE STRENGTH TO RISE ABOVE. TOGETHER, LET US FORGE A PATH FORWARD, KNOWING THAT THE HUMAN HEART IS RESILIENT, AND THAT THROUGH UNITY AND COMPASSION, WE CAN CREATE A WORLD FILLED WITH LOVE, HEALING, AND BOUNDLESS POSSIBILITIES.

LIGHT IN

SHADOWS

BY
VISHNU S KUMAR

www.ingramcontent.com/pod-product-compliance
Lightning Source LLC
Chambersburg PA
CBHW061338250726
48657CB00004B/1224